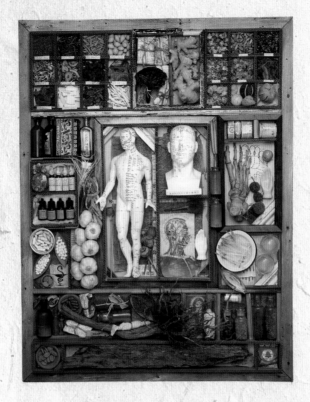

PRACTICAL
CHINESE
MEDICINE

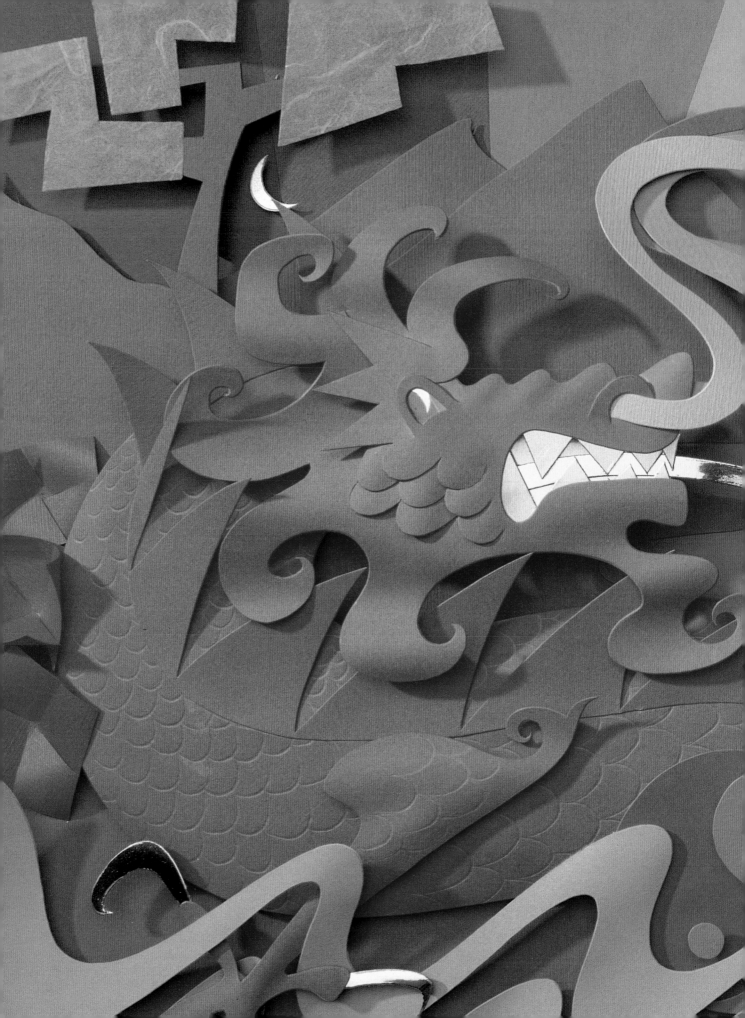

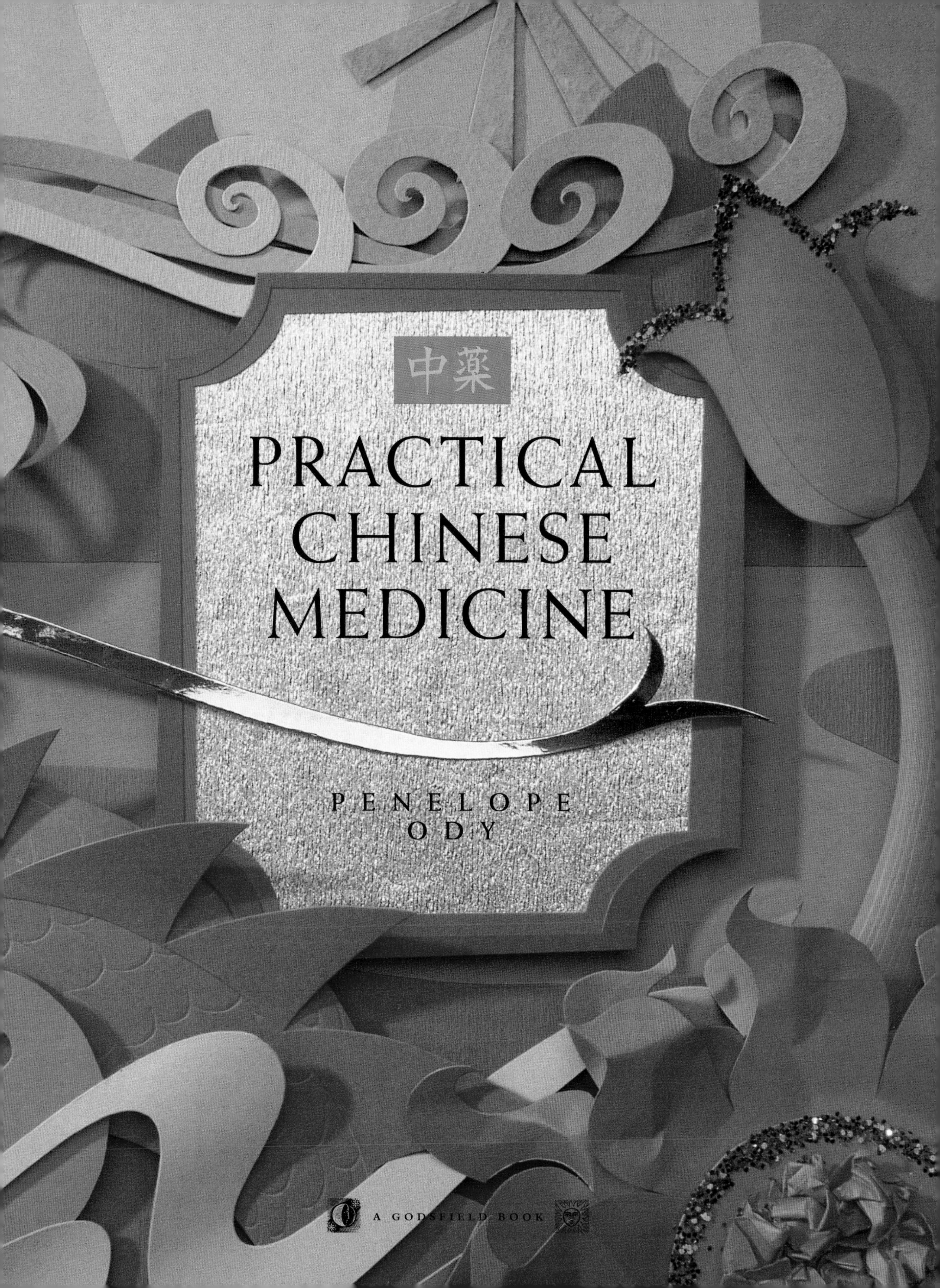

中藥

PRACTICAL
CHINESE
MEDICINE

P E N E L O P E
O D Y

A GODSFIELD BOOK

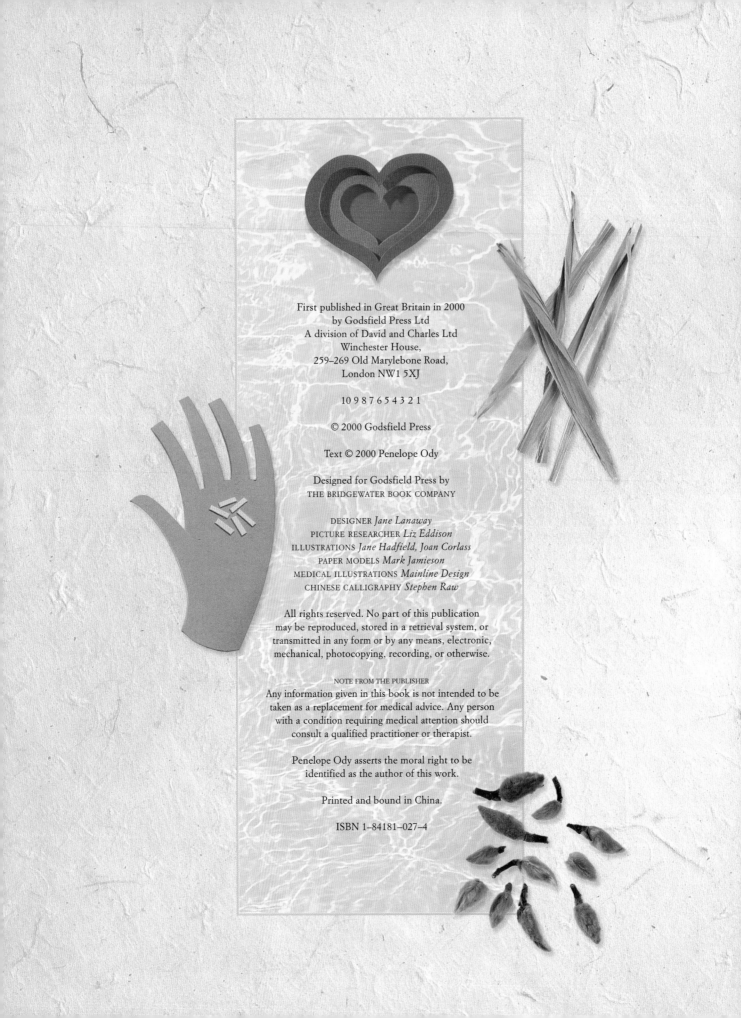

First published in Great Britain in 2000
by Godsfield Press Ltd
A division of David and Charles Ltd
Winchester House,
259–269 Old Marylebone Road,
London NW1 5XJ

10 9 8 7 6 5 4 3 2 1

© 2000 Godsfield Press

Text © 2000 Penelope Ody

Designed for Godsfield Press by
THE BRIDGEWATER BOOK COMPANY

DESIGNER *Jane Lanaway*
PICTURE RESEARCHER *Liz Eddison*
ILLUSTRATIONS *Jane Hadfield, Joan Corlass*
PAPER MODELS *Mark Jamieson*
MEDICAL ILLUSTRATIONS *Mainline Design*
CHINESE CALLIGRAPHY *Stephen Raw*

NOTE FROM THE PUBLISHER
Any information given in this book is not intended to be
taken as a replacement for medical advice. Any person
with a condition requiring medical attention should
consult a qualified practitioner or therapist.

Penelope Ody asserts the moral right to be
identified as the author of this work.

Printed and bound in China.

ISBN 1–84181–027–4

CONTENTS

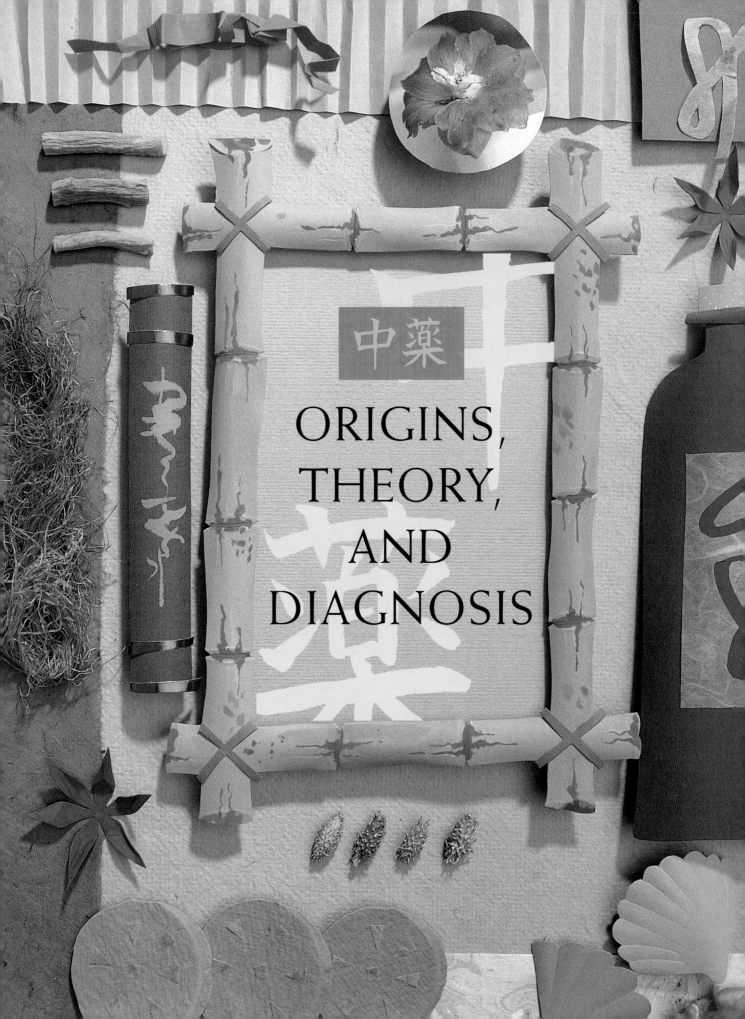

中薬

ORIGINS,
THEORY,
AND
DIAGNOSIS

HISTORY OF CHINESE MEDICINE

Like many traditional therapies, the origins of Chinese medicine are lost in the mists of time, with the discovery of herbs, medicine and healing attributed to three legendary emperors – a philosophical acupuncturist, a "divine farmer," and the Yellow Emperor.

ANCIENT BEGINNINGS

Long ago and far away, when the world began, lived the first mighty emperor, Fu Xi, who gave the Chinese a universal philosophy to interpret and explain all natural phenomena, and who reputedly made the first acupuncture needles.

Fu Xi was succeeded by Shen Nong, the "divine farmer," who first taught humankind how to cultivate grains and personally tasted hundreds of herbs to identify their healing properties.

The third ruler was Huang Di, the Yellow Emperor, the supreme ruler of the universe, who introduced music, medicine, mathematics, writing, and weapons.

Tradition says that these legendary figures lived some time between 4000 and 2500 BCE – and, although we now have no way of knowing whether they actually existed, their teachings were preserved and codified by later generations.

Fu Xi's *Ba Gua* of trigrams still forms the basis of the **I Ching**, used in divination and to guide decision taking. The **Shen Nong Ban Cao Jing** (**The Divine Farmer's Classic Herbal**) is the first of many famous collections detailing Chinese medicinal herbs still quoted today, while Huang Di's **Nei Jing Su Wen**

(**Canon of Internal Medicine**) – containing discussions on illness and diagnosis with his minister, Wu Peng – was the core textbook for Chinese physicians for generations.

Scholars generally date these early writings to around 400–500 BCE, although they are certainly based on much earlier traditions. The remedies and healing techniques they suggest are still used today: Shen Nong's **Herbal** recommends Chinese angelica root (*Dang Gui*) for regulating the menstrual cycle, and ephedra (*Ma Huang*) as a treatment for asthma. Today, doctors use the drug ephedrine, originally extracted from the herb, for a wide range of respiratory problems.

TAOIST ROOTS

In those days, China was predominantly Taoist. Taoism is a philosophy which recommends virtue as the ideal way to achieve prosperity, longevity, and immortality.

> 66 Medicines should co-ordinate in terms of yin and yang, like mother and child or brothers. 99
> *SHEN NONG BEN CAO JING*

Virtue meant conforming to nature and living in harmony with all things. This close association with the natural world is another important strand running through the Chinese approach to health and medicine that can readily be seen in the five-element model (*see* pages 12–13) and the important influence of yin and yang (*see* pages 10–11).

As in the West, there was no real understanding of human anatomy and physiology then, and very little surgery as we understand it today. Physicians could only use external information to guess at the inner workings of the body, and had no conception of microorganisms as a cause of disease.

Instead, in true Taoist fashion, they related illness and health to the environment – much as Hippocrates was doing in the West at around the same time – and saw disease in terms of external evils and internal imbalances in the flows of energy along channels or meridians (rather like our network of blood vessels) which they imagined in the body.

In the fourth century BCE, Qin Yueren – also known as Bian Que – was the first to set out the four diagnostic methods, which are still used by all Chinese practitioners today.

ALL SORTS OF THERAPIES

Although much of the earliest recorded Chinese medicine was herbal, we know that other treatment techniques, like acupuncture, have been used for just as long. Gold and silver needles have been found in tombs from the Han Dynasty (206 BCE–220 CE), while the **Nei Jing** identifies the various energy channels or meridians used in these treatments. The first recorded descriptions of acupuncture date from at least 1500 BCE, with many more detailed treatises surviving from the first century CE.

Other health routines date from a similar period: silk paintings discovered in Han tombs of the second century BCE show gymnastic movements that are remarkably similar to the *t'ai-chi* exercises familiar today (*see* pages 130–135). Another text, known as the **Zhuangzi**, dating from about 300 BCE, details the energizing effects of regular breathing exercises in what could be a description of *Qigong* (*see* pages 126–129).

AVOIDING INTERESTING TIMES

The traditional Chinese felt that change and transformation were to be avoided. For them, the traditional saying, "may you live in interesting times," is a curse, not a blessing.

So, for around five thousand years, Chinese culture continued in an established pattern with none of the dramatic upheavals of Western society – no major changes in religious faith, no waves of invading barbarians to overthrow the status quo, no real desire for exploration or trade beyond well-defined frontiers – only the survival of an extremely hierarchical and traditional society that slowly developed the beliefs and practices of its ancient, legendary founders.

ALL SORTS OF HERBS

The number of herbs in the Chinese repertoire grew steadily: 361 in Shen Nong's herbal; 730 in Tao Honjing's sixth-century new edition; 744 in the third great revision by Su Jing in 659 CE; and 1,746 in the **Zheng Lei Ben Cao** by Tang Shen-Wei in 1082.

The herbals contain more than just plants. The Chinese have always used mineral extracts and animal parts in their remedies. By 1578, when the herbalist Li Shi Zhen (1518–1583) produced **Compendium of Materia Medica** (**Ben Cao Gang Mu**), there were 1,892 vegetables, animals and minerals in regular use.

Li Shi Zhen, who also wrote the definitive text on pulse diagnosis, detailed 11,096 herbal formulas for use in specific syndromes.

In the 17th and 18th centuries, a spate of medical texts followed, such as the **Yizong Jinjian** (**Golden Mirror of Medicine**), which is still used in Chinese medical colleges. All followed the principles laid down by the Yellow Emperor, and reflected the five-element and yin–yang theories of the original Taoist teaching.

RIGHT **Chinese herbal remedies have always contained more than just plants. Treatments include mineral extracts and animal parts, as well as the cuttlefish and sea shells shown here.**

*Ze Xie
(water plantain)*

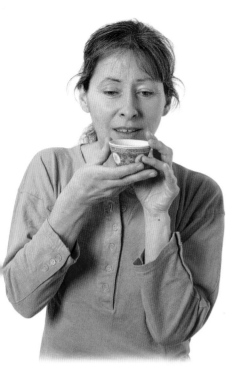

ABOVE **Tea drinking in China dates back to the days of Shen Nong, the husbandman who identified the healing uses of plants.**

FOLK TRADITIONS

The theories of the Yellow Emperor and Li Shi Zhen's thousands of remedies form just one style of Chinese medicine, and one that was largely confined to the affluent ruling classes. Chinese folk medicine – like folk medicine everywhere – was a much simpler affair, with household recipes handed down through families, and itinerant doctors, each specializing in a particular skill, wandering through the remote villages – just as in medieval Europe.

These wandering physicians were known as "bell doctors" for the bells that they traditionally rang to announce their arrival in a town. They used locally available herbs that were not always quite the same as the ones detailed in the classic herbals. Like folk healers everywhere, they used a combination of shamanism, herbal medicine, and ritual to effect their cures.

ENTER THE EUROPEANS

China's settled state of affairs was gradually eroded by the arrival of Europeans as China opened its doors to the West. Missionaries, from the 18th century onward, brought not only Christianity but Western-style medicine. The gaps in Chinese knowledge of anatomy and physiology were rudely exposed.

For example, dissection of corpses finally confirmed that there were not 24 holes in the lungs regulating breath control and that the heart had little to do with memory and thought, which was actually the preserve of a hitherto rather neglected organ called the brain.

Chinese doctors soon began to travel abroad to study – the first, Huang Kuan, arrived at Edinburgh University in the 1860s – and by the 1890s there was a College of Western Medicine in Hong Kong. By the time the first Chinese Republic was established in 1911, government ministers were actively trying to suppress traditional medicine in favor of a Western approach.

While the old "bell doctors" carried on practicing in rural China, traditional medical schools were banned and the classic medical texts dismissed as unscientific. Traditional medicine was largely kept alive by the *émigré* Chinese in Singapore, California, Hong Kong, and "Chinatowns" around the world.

CHANGE AND REVIVAL

In 1949, everything changed. The communists seized power, and improving public health became a key priority of theirs. New colleges of traditional Chinese medicine were established, along with a network of "barefoot doctors" who were trained in basic health skills and determined to improve the rudimentary health care facilities in the countryside. The old remedies were revived, too, by new pharmaceutical production plants set up to produce mass-market remedies for over-the-counter sale.

Today traditional medicine is readily available throughout China and thousands of newly qualified Chinese doctors have made their way to the West to fuel growing interest in the treatments in Europe and North America. At the same time, classic traditional Chinese formulae are being turned into mass-market products by Western drug companies.

THIS PAGE **Many familiar garden plants are important medicinal herbs.**

Bai Shao (white peony)

Xin Yi Hua (magnolia)

YIN AND YANG

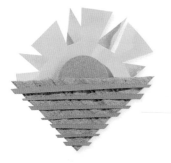

*T*he concepts of yin and yang are central to Chinese philosophy and underlie much of its traditional medicine; they can be difficult for the Western mind to comprehend. The concepts are closely intertwined and all things contain aspects of both of them.

TWO GREAT POWERS

To the ancient Taoists, yang and yin were the two great powers – the alternating aspects of the creative force central to all things. They were the light and dark sides of the mountain, the above and below, the outside and inside – paired and inseparable opposites.

Yang is sometimes described in the West as the more "masculine" aspect – in terms like movement, strength, outgoing, and active, while yin is couched in traditional feminine terms – such as static, frail, inward-looking, and passive. This is a rather artificial approach, as yin and yang are equal and contained in all things. What really decides masculinity or femininity is simply the balance between these two forces – their relative importance and activity.

Taoism is concerned with nature, the cosmos, and our relationship with our environment, so it is not surprising that yang and yin are most closely identified with, respectively, fire and water. For the Chinese, fire defines yang; anything that shares similar properties – things that are warm, bright, light, moving upward, active, or exciting – is regarded as yang. In contrast, water is cold, dim,

heavy, with a downward motion, passive, and inhibiting (or dampening); this describes yin.

Both aspects are, however, always present. While summer is more strongly yang, because it is a hot, bright season, it still contains some yin, and while damp and cold winter are more closely aligned with yin, it still contains an element of yang.

HEALTHY ASPECTS

The concept of yin and yang is applied in traditional Chinese medicine to the human body, so that substances (static things) are seen as more yin while functions (activities) are more yang.

Organs, blood, and body fluids tend to be yin, while the functions – transporting and transforming things, as with breathing and digestion – are seen as more yang.

Similarly, the exterior (outside) of the body is regarded as more yang, while the interior (inside) is more yin. The head (upward like fire) is yang. The feet (downward like water) are yin. Acupuncture meridians on the outer sides of the arms, legs, and back are yang, while those on the inner sides of the arms and legs, and across the abdomen, are yin.

The various organs of the body are classified as solid (*Zang*), which are more yin, or hollow (*Fu*), which are more yang in character – but they still contain both aspects. The Heart (a *Zang* organ) is predominantly yin, but it is in the upper half of the body, so it is rather more yang in character than the Liver (also *Zang* and yin), which is in the lower abdomen.

RELATIONSHIPS AND RESTRAINT

In a healthy body, the relationship between yin and yang is constantly changing: we take exercise and become more yang, or rest indoors and become more yin. These two energy forces also adapt and blend to our changing needs in what the Chinese refer to as "mutual restraint" – each controlling the other.

In disease and illness, this mutual restraint collapses and yin or yang get out of hand. Chinese medicine classifies four precise categories of yin–yang imbalance:
• overactive yin damaging yang
• overactive yang damaging yin
• excess yang resulting from a deficiency of yin
• excess yin resulting from a deficiency of yang.

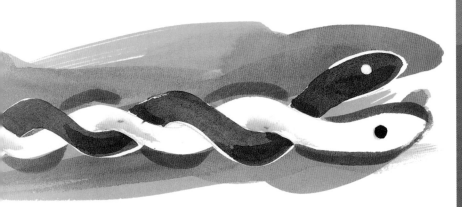

66 There is yang within yin and yin within yang. From dawn until noon, the yang of heaven is the yang within the yang. From noon until dusk, the yang of heaven is the yin within the yang. From dusk until midnight, the yin of heaven is the yin within the yin. From midnight until dawn, the yin of heaven is the yang within the yin. 99

HUANG DI NEI JING

Disease syndromes are defined in these terms. It is important to identify the nature of the imbalance to ensure accurate treatment. A disease characterized by fever and inflammation, for example, might be seen in terms of excessive yang. But that yang excess could be due to overactive yang, or to excess yang because yin is weak.

Treatment aimed at reducing or controlling yang might be appropriate if it is overactive, but if the problem is really yin deficiency, then restraining yang may simply serve to weaken the patient by reducing damaged energy levels still further.

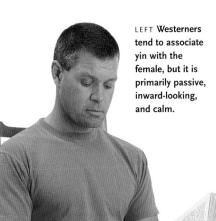

LEFT **Westerners tend to associate yin with the female, but it is primarily passive, inward-looking, and calm.**

RIGHT **Yang is active, outward-looking, and vigorous, and typified by heat and motion.**

CHARACTERISTICS OF YIN AND YANG

Yin	Yang
Water	Fire
Dark	Light
Cold	Hot
Passive	Active
Inside	Outside
Slow	Rapid
Right	Left
Dim	Bright
Downward	Upward
Substance	Function
Matter	Energy

FIVE ELEMENT THEORY

*W*hile early Western philosophers believed that the world was made up of four elements – earth, air, fire, and water, the Chinese conceived five primeval substances that were closely linked with the natural world they saw around them.

NATURAL PATTERNS

As early Chinese thinkers watched the changing seasons, they began to see a pattern emerging. Heavy winter rains caused new plants to emerge in the spring; these were scorched during the heat of high summer, leading to forest fires which created ashes, thus returning the plants to the earth – already known as the source of valuable metal ores. Metal surfaces conduct heat and so tend to be cold, thus causing water to condense, starting the cycle once more, with winter rains making the plants grow.

These observations developed into what is now known as the five-phase or five-element model. But the orderly Chinese mind did not limit this model to simple elements. Since all things in nature were one, then all things in nature must also conform to this model, and so a complex series of fives began to be associated with the five elements: five seasons, five directions, five colors, five solid body organs, five emotions, five tastes, five sounds, five smells – and so on.

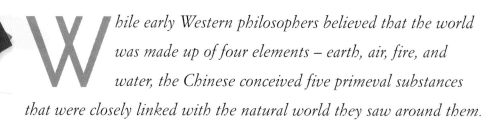

FIRE
Heart
Bitter

WOOD
Liver
Sour

EARTH
Spleen
Sweet

WATER
Kidney
Salty

METAL
Lung
Pungent

CHECKS AND CONTROLS

Just as the basic five elements interact with each other, so do their various characteristics. In the basic vision, Water promotes or gives rise to Wood, which promotes Fire, which gives rise to Earth, which promotes Metal, which leads back to Water. The Chinese see this as a "mother–son" relationship and say, for example, Water, the mother, gives birth to Wood, the son – and so on. The elements also have a controlling

function. This is again derived from observations: Water controls Fire, for example, while Fire will control Metal. Metal will chop Wood, which dominates the Earth beneath its roots, while Earth will soak up rain or divert rivers and so is Water's controlling element. In the reverse direction, these promoting and controlling tendencies act to restrain or weaken the same elements.

These cycles of promotion and control are essential to maintain balance and harmony: if any element becomes too strong and dominates the cycle, imbalance may follow, but the model ensures that this imbalance will eventually return to harmonious normality.

If Fire's control over Metal is excessive, for example, then Metal is weakened and becomes incapable of controlling Wood. Wood then grows too exuberant and starts to overcontrol Earth. Earth fails to check Water, which is overstrengthened and so exerts increased control on the overstrong Fire, which started the problem. Inevitably, if one element fails to fulfill its controlling/restraining duties, then the imbalance can become more severe and damaging.

h   *Metal*   *Water*   *Wood*

IMBALANCE AND DISEASE

Interaction between the five-phase groupings is an important aspect of traditional Chinese diagnosis and syndrome characterization. Thus, weakened Water (related to the Kidney) can fail to control Fire, which then attacks Metal (associated with the Lung) – which explains why, in some cases of, for example, asthma, a

ABOVE AND RIGHT   *Fire*
All things are derived from the five elements that govern not just matter, but emotions and seasonal change.

Chinese practitioner will declare that the Kidney is weak and prescribe suitable tonics rather than respiratory remedies.

> " With metal, wood is felled. With water, fire is extinguished. With wood, earth is rooted and loosened. With fire, metal is melted. And with earth, water is obstructed. This is the relationship among objects, too numerous to mention individually. "
>
> *HUANG DI NEI JING*

FIVE-PHASE ASSOCIATIONS

ELEMENT	Wood	Fire	Earth	Metal	Water
DIRECTION	East	South	Center	West	North
COLOR	Green	Red	Yellow	White	Black
SEASON	Spring	Summer	Late Summer *(traditionally from c. July 7 for a month)*	Fall	Winter
CLIMATE	Wind	Hot	Dampness	Dryness	Cold
SOLID ORGAN (*ZANG*)	Liver	Heart	Spleen	Lung	Kidney
HOLLOW ORGAN (*FU*)	Gall bladder	Small intestine	Stomach	Large intestine	Urinary bladder
SENSE ORGANS/ OPENINGS	Eyes/Sight	Tongue/Speech	Mouth/Taste	Nose/Smell	Ears/Hearing
EMOTION	Anger	Joy/Fright	Worry	Sadness/Grief	Fear
TASTE	Sour	Bitter	Sweet	Pungent/Acrid	Salty
TISSUES	Tendon	Blood vessels	Muscles	Skin	Bone
	Nails	Complexion	Lips	Body hair	Head hair
SOUND	Shouting	Laughing	Singing	Weeping	Groaning
SMELL	Rancid	Burned	Fragrant	Rotten	Putrid
BODY FLUID	Tears	Sweat	Saliva	Mucus	Urine
MEAT	Chicken	Mutton	Beef	Horse	Pork
CEREAL	Wheat	Glutinous millet	Millet	Rice	Beans

THE *ZANG* ORGANS

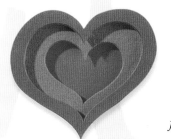

E arly Chinese physicians imagined five solid organs for the body, but the functions they suggested for each had little to do with what we now understand of their physiology. As well as physical functions, these organs are linked to emotional and spiritual factors.

SOLID ORGANS

In Chinese medicine, body functions are largely based on the five *Zang* organs – usually translated as viscera or solid organs: the Kidneys, Liver, Heart, Spleen, and Lungs. These body functions were derived from external observation rather than anatomical study and bear little relation to standard Western understanding. To make it clear that these theoretical functions are being discussed rather than actual organ pathology, it has become conventional in the West to give these Chinese "organ concepts" capital letters in order to differentiate them from Western ideas.

As well as being interlinked through their association with the five element model, the *Zang* organs each have a related "bowel" or hollow organ (the *Fu* organs, *see* pages 18–19) and are connected to these by meridians or acupuncture channels.

These organs are part of a complex network involving five fundamental substances (*see* pages 22–27). They are affected not only by the strength or weakness of their immediate neighbors in the five-phase model, but also by these fundamental substances. Each one also has very specific functions.

HEART

- Controls mental activities
- Governs the Blood circulation and vessels
- Is seen in the complexion
- Is linked to the tongue.

The Heart is said to be the ruling member of the *Zang–Fu* organs, and controls all life processes. This approach is similar to other traditional medical theories – including Ayurveda and ancient Egyptian belief – where the heart is closely associated with the soul and emotions.

In Chinese medicine, the Heart, rather than the brain is seen as controlling "mental activities" – which the Chinese understand as meaning a wide range of thought processes, perception, and mental health. In contrast, the brain is regarded simply as a system for receiving and storing information, with no real involvement in thought processes.

Mental disorder is believed to be caused by some sort of damage to the Heart. Remedies which are traditionally said to "calm the spirit" are often those which, in Western terms, would be used to regulate heart activity.

The Heart also, and not surprisingly, is described as governing

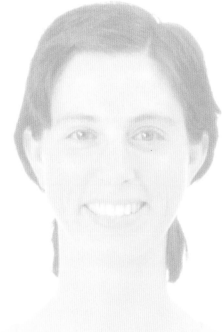

Blood and blood vessels. When the Heart's energy (*Qi*) is strong, the Blood is vigorous, and the person will be healthy and full of life.

This close association with blood vessels means that the health of the Heart is mirrored in the face. If Heart *Qi* is strong, the complexion is ruddy and healthy; if the *Qi* is weak, then the face is pale. The Heart is also associated with the tongue in the five-element model, so the Chinese argue that taste is a reflection of Heart *Qi* vitality.

SPLEEN

- Controls digestion
- Controls the limbs and flesh
- Keeps Blood in the vessels
- Stores intention or determination
- Linked to the mouth/appetite and reflected in the lips.

The concept of the Spleen is quite difficult for Westerners to grasp. For Westerners, the Spleen is a rather vague organ that has something to do with disposing of old red blood cells. So the Chinese view of the Spleen as central to digestion and muscle development comes as something of a surprise.

The Spleen is traditionally believed to absorb nutrients from food and then to stimulate the dispersal of this "food essence" throughout the body. If Spleen *Qi* is strong, this works well and the body is healthy. If it is weak, then tissues become malnourished.

The Spleen performs the same function with water extracted from food, sending it through the body to reach the Kidneys.

This association with nutrition also explains why the Spleen is responsible for building strong limbs and well-developed muscles.

The muscles are linked with the mouth and lips, so these are said to reflect the condition of the Spleen. Healthy pink lips suggest good nutrition and strong Spleen *Qi*. Pale lips, and upsets in taste or appetite, are associated with weakened Spleen.

Strong Spleen *Qi* is also needed to keep Blood flowing in the vessels,

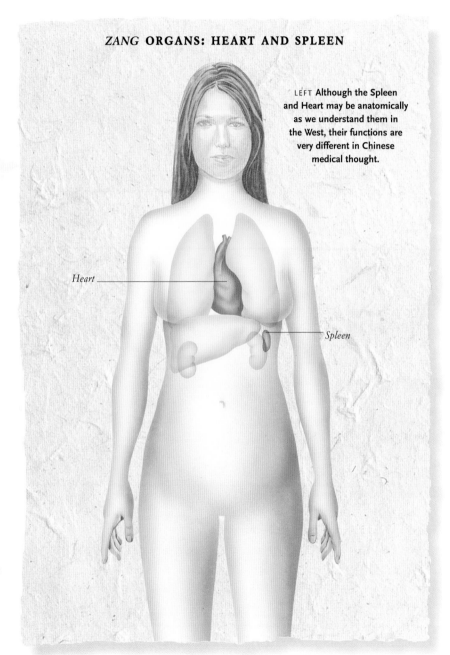

ZANG ORGANS: HEART AND SPLEEN

LEFT **Although the Spleen and Heart may be anatomically as we understand them in the West, their functions are very different in Chinese medical thought.**

Heart

Spleen

but if it is weak, then there may be hemorrhages or subcutaneous bleeding as a result.

Like the Heart and other organs, the Spleen is involved in mental activities and is specifically responsible for *Yi*, which has variously been translated as intention, willpower, determination, or an awareness of the possibilities that are open to us to make changes in our lives.

LUNGS

- Control *Qi* and respiration
- Maintain the downward flow of Fluid, regulate Water circulation
- Store vitality or "animal energy"
- Are linked to the nose
- *Qi* is reflected in the skin and hair.

While Chinese medicine regards the Lungs as responsible for respiration, the breath is also closely associated with vital energy.

Breath as energy is familiar to Westerners from exercise disciplines like yoga and *Qigong*, so the Chinese assertion that the "Lungs control *Qi*" appears logical. *Qi* is subdivided into many different categories (*see* pages 22–27), and the Lungs are particularly associated with "defense *Qi*" (*Wei Qi*), which they help to send to the body's surface in order to repel invading evils which may cause imbalance and ill-health.

Lung *Qi* also tends to move downward, so it encourages the flow of Water and Fluids through the body to the Kidney and Urinary Bladder. Lung problems can thus be blamed for edema and fluid retention in Chinese medicine.

The Lungs' aspect of mental activity (*Po*) may be translated as "vitality" and is associated more with the physical side of concentration rather than thought processes.

The Lungs are connected with the nose and sense of smell, while their connection with *Wei Qi* and surface energies highlights the view that Lung *Qi* is seen in the skin and body hair. Healthy skin shows strong Lung *Qi*.

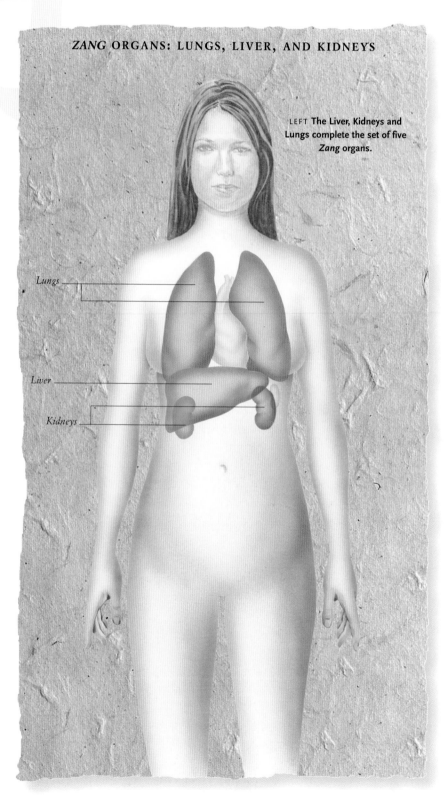

ZANG ORGANS: LUNGS, LIVER, AND KIDNEYS

LEFT **The Liver, Kidneys and Lungs complete the set of five** *Zang* **organs.**

Lungs

Liver

Kidneys

KIDNEYS

- Regulate Water in the body
- Coordinate respiration
- Store vital essence (*Jing*)
- Produce bone marrow
- Store determination
- Are linked to the ears and genitals
- *Qi* is seen in the hair.

The Kidneys are, understandably, closely associated with water metabolism and regulation – as such, they are linked to the Lungs so take their share in the respiration process. Chinese medicine associates water regulation with "Body Fluids." These are divided into "clear fluid," which circulates through the organs and tissues, and "turbid fluid," which is transformed into sweat and urine and is excreted. The Kidneys send the clear fluid upward and the turbid fluid downward for disposal. The Kidneys also help to direct the *Qi* flow downward, so helping the work of the Lungs during inhalation. If Kidney *Qi* is weak, it can lead to breathing problems and certain types of asthma.

The Kidneys are also important in storing vital essence or *Jing* (*see* pages 22–27). Part of this *Jing* can be transformed into Kidney *Qi*, which also affects our energy and aging processes.

Traditional theory maintains that the vital essence stored in the Kidneys is transformed into bone marrow that spreads along the spinal cord to the brain – itself originally believed to be made of bone marrow. Through this connection with the bones and brain,

the Kidneys are also associated with head hair. An abundance of lustrous hair is believed to indicate healthy Kidney *Qi*, and thus strong essence and creativity.

Kidney *Qi*'s association with the reproductive system links the Kidneys to the outward genitalia.

LIVER

- Stores Blood
- Regulates the flow of *Qi*
- Stores the soul
- Controls the tendons
- Can be seen in the nails
- Is linked to the eyes.

While the Heart governs the Blood flow, the Liver is said to store Blood and regulate its release into the body as needed. This helps to explain why the Chinese associate the Liver with the female menstrual cycle and will often treat gynecological problems with Liver tonics.

The Liver regulates "*Qi* flow" – or the way this vital energy circulates through our bodies. The ideal is for a smooth and constant flow of *Qi* with no stagnation (which, in Chinese theory, will lead to dysfunction). Acupuncture treatments generally are designed to stimulate *Qi* flow and to dispel stagnation.

The Liver also is said to "store the soul," which is a rather strange concept for the Western mind. In Chinese medicine, the "spirit" is a complex concept, combining mental activity, consciousness, determination, "*Po*" (a rather untranslatable entity meaning a more body-centered aspect

of soul, sometimes defined as vitality and associated with the Lungs), and an ethereal aspect of soul called *Hun*, which equates more with the concept of soul familiar to Westerners. *Hun* is stored in the Liver.

In the Taoist world view, calmness and tranquillity – along with a tendency to watch and wait rather than to actively interfere with events, are important. So, maintaining a calm soul – by ensuring a smooth flow of *Qi* through the liver – is essential for good health and longevity.

In the five-phase model the Liver is also associated with the tendons, eyes, and nails. Aching tendons, generally most noticeable in the knees, can thus suggest Liver imbalance, while strong, healthy pink nails suggest good Liver *Qi*. Poor eyesight is seen as a result of deficient Liver Blood, while irritant conditions like conjunctivitis are defined in terms of Heat or Wind affecting the Liver or Liver meridians.

BELOW **The health of the Liver is reflected in the health of the nails. Strong, healthy nails suggest the Liver is also in good condition.**

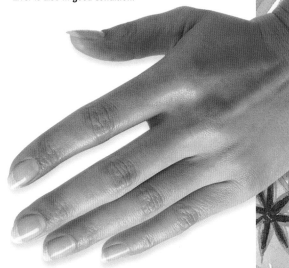

THE *FU* ORGANS

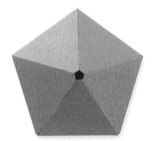

Each solid organ has an associated hollow organ or "bowel" which is linked via the meridians. The five Fu organs are the Small Intestine, Stomach, Large Intestine, Urinary Bladder, and Gall Bladder, which each form a Zang Fu pair with one of the solid organs.

SMALL INTESTINE

The Small Intestine is paired with the Heart and is believed to "receive and contain" water and food. It is said to convert them into useful substances – much as it does in conventional Western physiology.

The Small Intestine also sends the unusable materials onward for excretion. Chinese medicine usually describes these usable and unusable materials as "clear" and "turbid." Excess Heat or Damp in the system can increase the turbidity and be related to subsequent urinary problems.

STOMACH

The Stomach is paired with the Spleen; it takes in and digests food and is regarded in Chinese theory as a reservoir for food and water. Its effectiveness in starting the digestive process is seen as a function of stomach *Qi*. If it is strong, then the food is propelled onward to the small intestine; if it is weak, then food tends to stagnate in the stomach.

Spleen and Stomach are very closely associated, more so than the other *Zang Fu* pairings. The two terms are sometimes used interchangeably.

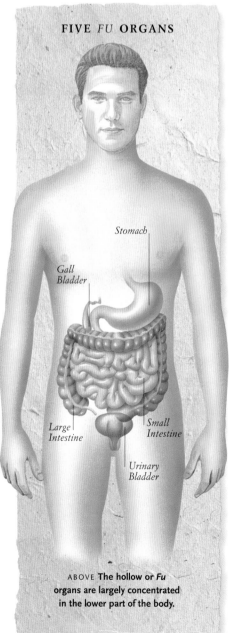

FIVE *FU* ORGANS

Stomach

Gall
Bladder

Large
Intestine

Small
Intestine

Urinary
Bladder

ABOVE **The hollow or *Fu*
organs are largely concentrated
in the lower part of the body.**

Importantly, Stomach *Qi* is always slightly turbid or damp, as it is involved in sending nutrients and waste materials downward, while Spleen *Qi* is always clear, since it is involved in the upward transportation of water and has an aversion to dampness.

LARGE INTESTINE

The Large Intestine is associated with the Lungs. Like the other *Fu* organs, it is mainly involved with transport and transformation. It is involved in compacting the solid wastes from our food, so the Chinese describe it as "governing body fluid."

If the Large Intestine fails to reabsorb sufficient moisture, then stools are going to be watery and there is going to be diarrhea. Blockages in the Large Intestine – as in constipation – are believed to interfere with the descending function of Lung *Qi*.

URINARY BLADDER

The Urinary Bladder is paired with the Kidney and, conventionally, has the job of storing and discharging urine. The Kidney separates the "clear" (usable) fluid from the unusable "turbid" component, so the

Urinary Bladder is another organ largely involved in transporting turbid materials away from the body.

Urinary activity is said to be controlled by Kidney yang – if this is weak, then problems like nocturia and frequent micturition can follow. The Chinese compare this aspect of Kidney energy to "the fire on the wok," which, when strong, will "evaporate" the urine – thus overcoming a need for frequent urination.

GALL BLADDER

This is paired with the Liver and, as in conventional medicine, is regarded as a reservoir for bile. Chinese theory, however, regards bile not as a breakdown product from digestion, but as surplus Liver *Qi.*

The Gall Bladder is associated with decisiveness, activity, and decision-making. A common idiomatic expression for a vigorous or particularly brave person is to say that they have "a big gall bladder."

If Gall Bladder energy is weak, then the person tends to be a ditherer and finds decision-making difficult. Together with the Liver, the Gall Bladder is also involved in ensuring a smooth flow of *Qi* and blood.

SAN JIAO

Chinese medicine also talks of a sixth *Fu* organ: the "triple burner" or *San Jiao.* This is a concept dating back to the Yellow Emperor and is an attempt to describe the body's digestive function. The *San Jiao* is sometimes represented as a kind of formless sewage system which transports and transforms nutrients while eliminating waste material. Other early texts suggest that it supports various kinds of *Qi.*

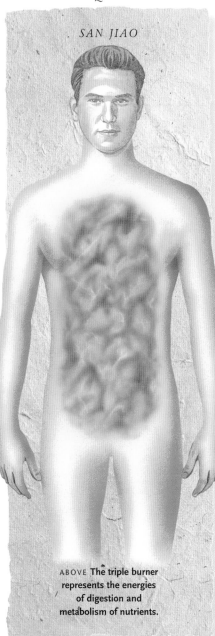

SAN JIAO

ABOVE **The triple burner represents the energies of digestion and metabolism of nutrients.**

The *San Jiao* can be a difficult concept for Westerners and is perhaps best regarded as a generalization of internal functions related to regulation and digestion. It has three components:
• The Upper *Jiao*, which relates to the chest above the diaphragm. It is associated with the generalized function of Heart and Lungs.
• The Middle *Jiao*, between diaphragm and navel, which reflects the functions of Spleen and Stomach.
• The Lower *Jiao*, below the navel, which is associated with the functions of Kidney and Urinary Bladder.

The *San Jiao* is important in acupuncture and is connected to its own paired organ, the Pericardium (the sac around the heart) – which the tidy-minded sometimes add to the list of *Zang* organs, although the classic Chinese texts tend to see the Pericardium–triple burner pairing as a subset of the Small Intestine.

EXTRAORDINARY ORGANS

Six other body "organs" are known as the miscellaneous or extraordinary organs, or "organs of consciousness," because they are all associated with "essence" (*Jing*). These are Brain, Bone Marrow, Blood Vessels, Uterus, Channels or meridians, and – rather confusingly – the Gall Bladder, which comes into both categories because it is associated with mental activities.

THE SEVEN EMOTIONS

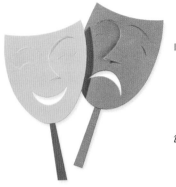

The five-phase model links a particular emotion with each of the elements and Zang Fu organs. These emotions make up the classic "Seven Emotions" (Lung and Heart each have two); when in excess, they are seen as causes of disease and ill-health.

JOY

This emotion is linked to the Heart and to the Western mind is a cheerful, positive concept that we find difficult to see as damaging. The positive side of Joy seen in these terms is beneficial.

Traditional Chinese society was, however, excessively hierarchical and deeply conservative, so Joy seen in terms of overexuberance and inappropriate behavior is damaging. We can perhaps imagine "Joy" as a rowdy group of excited teenagers yelling noisily in the street and upsetting elderly passers-by, rather than the happy sense of contentment and light-heartedness associated with the word in the West.

This "inappropriateness" is the negative aspect of Joy and too much of it will damage the Heart and also the Lungs which are located close by in the Upper *Jiao*.

Too much Joy damaging Heart *Qi* can lead to an inability to concentrate, while the sort of hysterical laughter associated with some forms of mental disorder is also associated by the Chinese with damaged Heart *Qi*.

FRIGHT

Panic or sudden fear from some dramatic external event is also associated with the Heart. This association can be easily understood in the West; its symptoms are "panic attacks," with their palpitations, mental restlessness, and cold sweats. In Chinese medicine, fright is said to send the Heart *Qi* "wandering about, adhering to nothing."

WORRY

The emotion linked to the Spleen is usually described as "pensiveness," worry, or "overthinking" – that is, dwelling too much on a particular problem, or concentrating too hard for too long.

The result is stagnation of Spleen *Qi*, which in Chinese theory manifests as depression, anxiety, poor appetite, weakened limbs, abdominal bloating, and, in women, menstrual irregularities.

Pensiveness is said to originate in the Heart, so an excess can damage Heart *Qi*. A common syndrome associated with excess worry is described as "depressed Heat in the Heart and Spleen," which can involve insomnia, palpitations, and constipation.

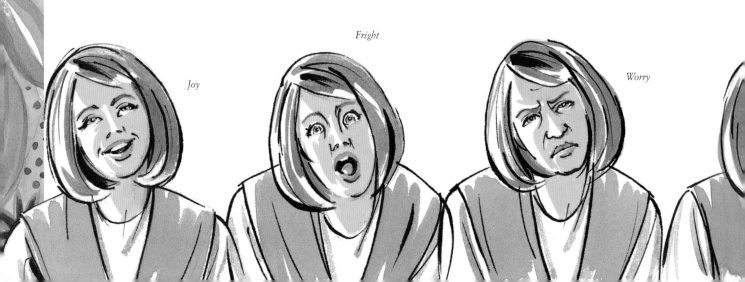

Fright

Joy

Worry

SADNESS

Sadness is linked to the Lungs, and an excess is considered to "consume Lung *Qi*" and also to lead to respiratory problems as well as cause stagnation. This may then affect the vitality of associated organs (following the five-element relationship).

Sadness affecting the lungs is very common and may be observed as bronchitis and asthmatic problems, for example. They frequently seem to follow bereavement, while chesty coughs are common in those who are unhappy.

GRIEF

Extreme grief or shock is also linked to the Lungs and, since the Lungs are responsible for *Qi* circulation, severe shock affects the entire body. Symptoms include those associated with "shock" in the West – pallor, breathing problems, and a sense of suffocation in the chest, as well as loss of appetite, constipation, and urinary problems.

FEAR

Fear is linked to the Kidneys. An excess will reverse the normal, upward flow of Kidney *Qi*, leading to listlessness, lower back pains, urinary problems, and a desire for solitude. Bedwetting in children can be explained in these terms, with timidity and shyness often being associated symptoms. In women, fear damages the Kidney and can also cause irregular menstruation.

ANGER

In Chinese medicine, the Liver is associated with Anger. Too much makes Liver *Qi* rise, leading to headaches, flushed face, dizziness, and red eyes.

In the West, the liver is traditionally associated with strong emotions – notably love and bravery. Westerners have absorbed some of the Chinese imagery for this in the term *gung-ho*, with its association of excess activity and military aggression. It is said to derive from the Chinese word for "Liver Fire."

> The emotions of joy and anger are injurious to the spirit. Cold and heat are injurious to the body. Violent anger is hurtful to yin; violent joy is hurtful to yang. When rebellious emotions rise to heaven, the pulse expires and leaves the body. When joy and anger are without moderation, then cold and heat exceed all measure and life is no longer secure.
>
> *HUANG DI NEI JING*

BELOW **The seven emotions ranging from joy to anger are believed to affect our physical well-being and general health.**

Fear

Anger

Sadness

Grief

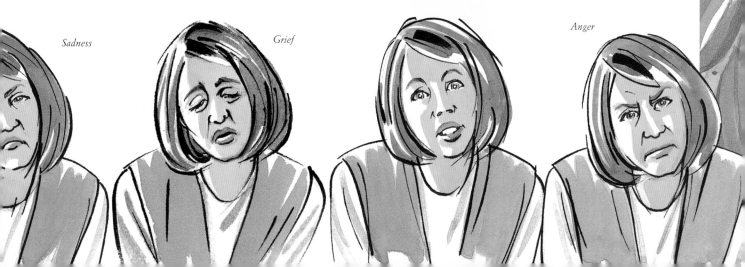

FUNDAMENTAL SUBSTANCES

Chinese medicine talks of "life materials" or "fundamental substances" – concepts that are different from the Western view of physical entities. Westerners may find the concepts of Qi (as a "vital energy") and Blood easy to understand, but other "life materials" may be more difficult to grasp.

JING

Although *Qi* is more familiar to Westerners, for the Chinese, *Jing* or "essence" is even more important. It is *the* fundamental substance – being the source of living organisms and the most important of this group of life materials.

Jing is stored in the Kidneys and comes in two forms. First is the congenital, parental, or innate essence – this is with us from birth, and we inherit it from our parents. It is also known as "reproductive essence" or "before heaven" and controls both reproduction and creativity. The second type is the acquired essence, which is produced by the Spleen from food, air, and water; it is known as "after heaven" and reflects the quality

BELOW **Good diet and healthy living will help add to our innate store of *Jing*.**

BELOW **The congenital form of *Jing* is with us from birth.**

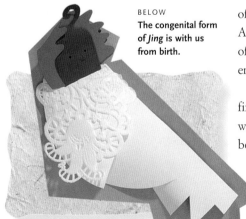

of your nutrition and lifestyle. Although quite separate, the two types of essence are interdependent and can encourage each other.

Our store of congenital essence is fixed – we cannot add to what we were born with and it will, gradually, become depleted over a lifetime. Its loss is associated with the physical signs of aging, such as graying hair and hearing problems.

Acquired essence is, however, continually being replenished from what we eat. So a healthy, balanced diet can build this sort of essence and in some ways compensate for any weaknesses in inherited *Jing.*

Jing is essential for reproduction. The gradual erosion of our congenital essence is characterized, in women, by an end to childbearing abilities and the menopause, which tends to be treated as a Kidney weakness problem.

RIGHT **Excesses and over-activity will erode *Jing* at any age of your life.**

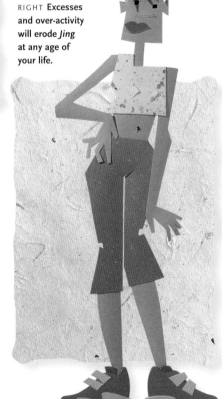

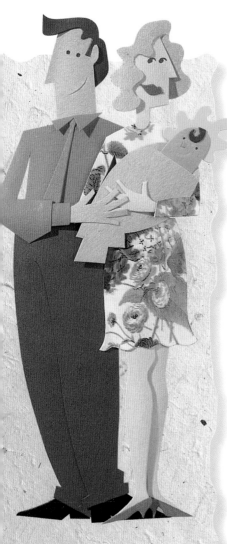

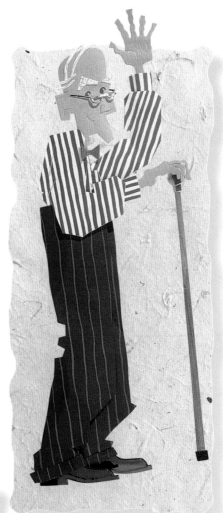

innate creativity. It makes sense – in Chinese medicine at least – that creative geniuses often rapidly exhaust their *Jing* and die, as Mozart is believed to have done, from Kidney failure.

The link with bone marrow explains why *Jing* is said to nourish the Blood. So, problems associated with Blood deficiency may actually be cases of *Jing* deficiency.

Just as with the five-element relationship of the *Zang Fu* organs, Chinese physicians are always

RIGHT **Problems with conception and miscarriage may be related to *Jing* weakness.**

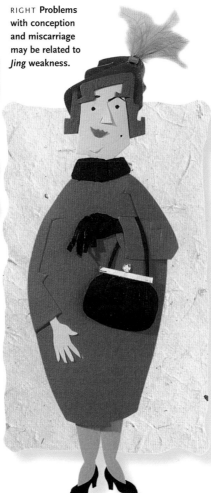

ABOVE **The gray hair and hearing problems of old age are related to declining Kidney energy.**

Essence can also change its form and feed some of the other life materials. It is interchangeable with Blood and can be converted into *Qi*. *Qi* also will strengthen the Spleen; thus, indirectly, it can help to strengthen the formation of acquired essence.

Jing also is believed to produce bone marrow, which practitioners of Chinese medicine associate with the brain (often described as the "sea of the marrow"), so it is not surprising that *Jing* tends to be associated with

looking for these interactions when trying to identify the cause of disease or ill health.

Poor memory, lack of concentration, or any sort of brain damage, for example, might be blamed on a weakness in bone marrow due to *Jing* deficiency and be treated with Kidney tonics. The same applies to reproductive problems such as impotence or miscarriage.

LEFT **The menopause is explained in Chinese medicine in terms of *Jing* weakness – *Jing* is vital for reproduction.**

Qi

Qi – often understood in the West as our inner energy level – actually comes in a wide variety of types. Its main characteristic is motion: the activity of life.

There are many subdivisions of *Qi* and the names used to categorize these numerous varieties can be confusing. Some scholars suggest that as many as 32 different varieties of *Qi*, each with its own specific function and characteristics, have been described in Chinese texts over the past 2,500 years, with changing emphases and terminology over the centuries adding to the confusion.

Basically, *Qi*, like essence, is a mixture of energies derived from the food we eat and the air we breathe, plus an element inherited from our parents which is with us from birth. These raw ingredients then combine and are transformed in a variety of ways to make the different sorts of *Qi* that circulate in the body.

As well as these various subgroups, *Qi* is also seen as actual activity, that is, the physiological function of the various body organs. Heart *Qi*, for example, is the action of the Heart – not just an immaterial sort of energy state. Saying that "Spleen *Qi* is deficient," for example, can indicate that digestive function is weak, while blockages in the channel *Qi* (which flows through the acupuncture meridians, *see* pages 28–31) can lead to pain and discomfort.

DIFFERENT SORTS OF *QI*

• Primordial or *Yuan Qi*, like the congenital essence, from which it derives, is with us from birth and is essential for producing new life. This sort of *Qi* provides the basic energy for the *Zang Fu* organs and can be transformed into any of the other main types of *Qi* as required. It is stored in the lower back, which is called the "gate of life" in Chinese medicine.

• Pectoral or *Zong Qi* is stored in the chest and derives from a mixture of "grain *Qi*" (*Gu Qi*), that is produced from food by the spleen, and "nature *Qi*" (*Kong Qi*), which derives from the air we breathe. Among its various functions, pectoral *Qi* fuels the circulation of Blood and regulates heartbeat.

• Normal or upright *Qi* (*Zheng Qi*) is the term generally used to describe most of the body's *Qi*. This is derived from a mixture of the primordial, grain, and nature *Qi*, which spreads through the entire body. *Zheng Qi* is referred to when one talks of the "*Qi*" of particular *Zang Fu* organs; it warms and invigorates the body, keeps Blood and Body Fluids in their appropriate channels, and can be subdivided into many other categories and functions.

BELOW **Primordial *Qi*, or *Yuan Qi*, is with us from birth, like the congenital essence. It is vital for producing new life.**

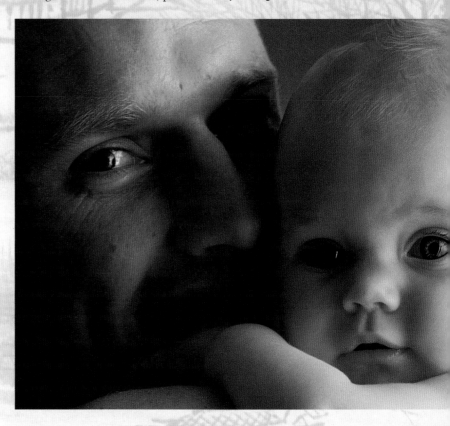

• Nourishing *Qi* (*Ying Qi*) is largely produced from the grain *Qi* of our food, which is collected and transformed in the Spleen. It flows through the blood vessels, becoming part of the Blood, and supplying nutrients throughout the body. In cases of "Blood deficiency," a Chinese physician will try to strengthen this nourishing *Qi*.

• Defensive *Qi* (*Wei Qi*), which protects the body is sometimes equated in Chinese medicine with the Western concept of the immune system. It is also partly derived from the grain *Qi* and can be regarded as an aspect of normal *Qi*. In Chinese medicine, poor health is often blamed

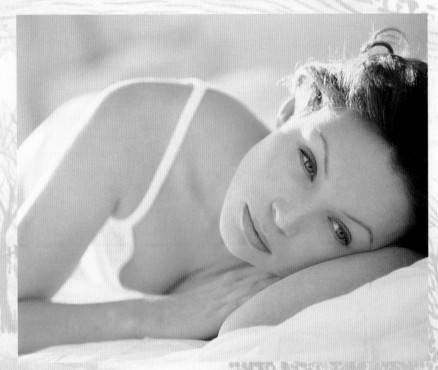

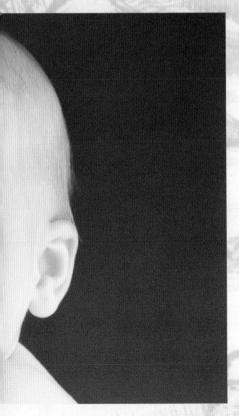

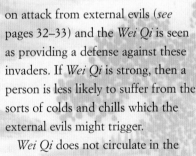

on attack from external evils (*see* pages 32–33) and the *Wei Qi* is seen as providing a defense against these invaders. If *Wei Qi* is strong, then a person is less likely to suffer from the sorts of colds and chills which the external evils might trigger.

Wei Qi does not circulate in the Blood or channels, but travels through the skin and muscles, where it controls the opening and closing of pores to regulate body temperature and moisten the skin.

Circulating *Wei Qi* tends to be a daytime phenomenon – traveling up the spine and across the head in the morning, then down the front of the body during the afternoon to reach the lower spine at night, where it retreats back into the body.

ABOVE **Imbalance in the *Wei Qi* can be a cause of insomnia, as its internal movement will disturb the body at night.**

Therefore the time of any external injury is regarded as highly significant in Chinese medicine. A head injury in the morning, for example, is likely to have damaged the circulating *Wei Qi,* and so will be harder to treat than a head injury later in the day when the *Wei Qi* is elsewhere.

Imbalance in the *Wei Qi* can be a cause of insomnia (as its internal movement will disturb the body at night). It is also linked to skin disease, since that is where it is most often found. Dry and itchy skin, for example, can be a sign of *Wei Qi* deficiency.

BLOOD

Blood or *Xue* is a rather more tangible entity than *Qi* and is formed from a mixture of nourishing *Qi,* food essence, and Body Fluids. It is the familiar red stuff circulating in our blood vessels that transports nutrients throughout the body.

Inevitably, the Chinese concept of "Blood" goes a little further. It is regarded as essential for mental activities. If Blood and *Qi* are strong, a person will be clear-thinking and vigorous; if not, that person may have problems concentrating.

Because of the link with Body Fluids, sweating is seen as something which can damage Blood and lead to deficiency. Since the Liver stores Blood, any damage to the Liver is likely to harm Blood, with weak Liver *Qi* leading to Blood stagnation.

BODY FLUIDS

The Chinese tend to describe any internal liquid as "Fluid," or *Jin–Ye,* with *Jin* indicating the clear aspect of fluid and *Ye* suggesting the turbid component. Among the Body Fluids are substances like saliva, gastric juices, phlegm, tears, mucus, and sweat. Body Fluids are seen as derived from our food and water, and are converted in the Spleen and Stomach into the *Jin* and *Ye.*

Jin Fluids are carried partly in the Blood and also manifest as sweat. The thicker *Ye* Fluid nourishes the inner parts of the body such as joints, body orifices, brain, and bone marrow.

Both Blood and Body Fluids are regarded as predominantly yin in nature, so any illness involving dryness or a lack of sweating might be seen as involving yin deficiency.

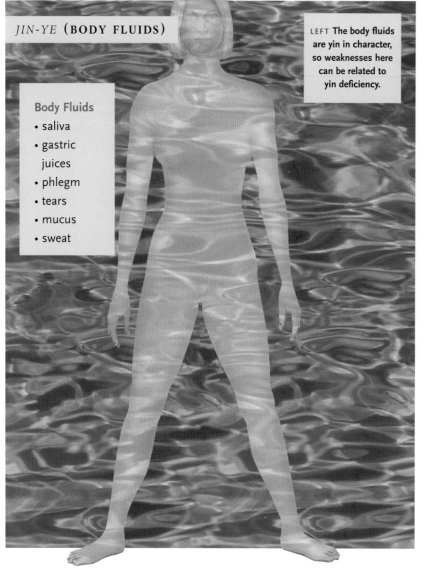

JIN-YE (BODY FLUIDS)

Body Fluids
- saliva
- gastric juices
- phlegm
- tears
- mucus
- sweat

LEFT The body fluids are yin in character, so weaknesses here can be related to yin deficiency.

BELOW The Taoists saw physical and spiritual aspects as inseparable and closely aligned to the natural rhythm of the world around us.

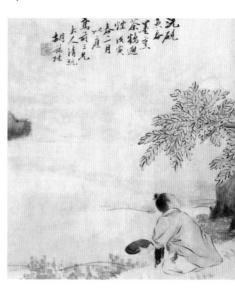

Like *Qi* and Blood, the *Jin–Ye* circulate through the body – largely under the control of the Spleen, Lungs, and Kidneys. So weaknesses in any of these organs might be blamed for a resulting Body Fluid deficiency or dysfunction.

SHEN

The final life material is even more nebulous than *Jing* or *Qi*. *Shen* is generally translated as "spirit" – the inner strength behind both essence and energy that is closely associated with human consciousness.

Shen is sometimes described as "awareness" – the alertness that can be seen in the bright eyes of someone who is fully conscious of their surroundings, actions, and capabilities. *Shen* is also closely linked to lifestyle and creativity.

RIGHT **Bright eyes and an intrinsic alertness characterize *Shen*, which, in Chinese medicine, is translated as "spirit" or "awareness."**

If *Shen* is damaged in any way, then the person may be forgetful, slow-thinking, suffer from insomnia, or – in extreme cases – be violent and deranged. People who behave erratically or jump from one subject to another in conversation are often suffering from some form of *Shen* disharmony. *Jing*, *Qi*, and *Shen* are referred to in Chinese tradition as "the three treasures."

For the past three hundred years or so, the "spiritual" and "physical" aspects of life have tended to be divided in the West into two quite separate categories. This idea usually is said to have originated with the French philosopher René Descartes (1596–1650 CE), who argued that intangibles like religious faith have no place in the physical world.

Chinese medicine, however, is still firmly rooted in the beliefs of the early Taoists, where the physical and spiritual are inseparable and part of the total unity of the cosmos.

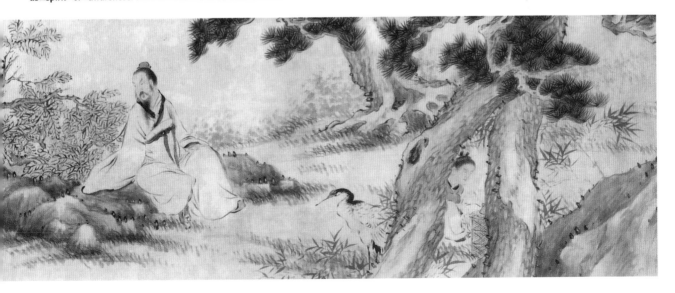

THE MERIDIANS

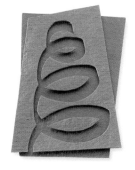

*I*n traditional Chinese, theory the meridians – or channels – are seen as a network of conduits which carry and distribute Qi to all parts of the body. When this flow of vital energy is disrupted, disease and poor health follow; acupuncture evolved as a way of keeping channels open and energy flowing.

MERIDIANS AND ACU POINTS

The complex web of energy meridians is unique and central to Chinese medical theory. The idea of three-dimensional channels running through the body, just as our visible nerves and blood vessels do, goes back to the days of the Yellow Emperor, while the first recorded descriptions of acupuncture to treat disease date to the Shang dynasty of about 1500 BCE.

Just as with emotions, fluids and other parts of the body, this mesh of channels is linked to each of the ten *Zang* and *Fu* organs, as well as the Pericardium and *San Jiao* (*see* pages 18–19). This gives twelve main or regular channels – collectively known as *Jing Mai* – which may be yin or yang in character, depending on whether they are associated with *Zang* or *Fu* organs. In addition, there is a group of eight "extraordinary channels" with very specific functions.

Each of the twelve regular channels has a collateral, with an additional one assigned to the Spleen, and one each for the two most important extraordinary channels – the *Ren Mai* and *Du Mai* (*see* pages 30–31). This gives fifteen minor channels or collaterals (*Luo Mai*) that are smaller and spread out from the main channels, connecting each yin/yang pair.

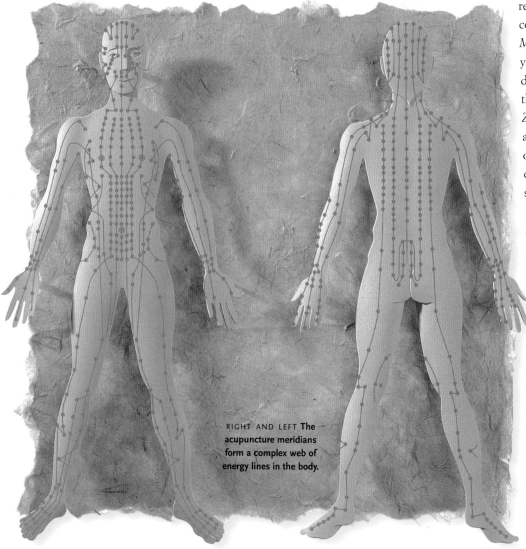

RIGHT AND LEFT **The acupuncture meridians form a complex web of energy lines in the body.**

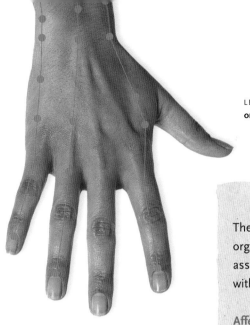

LEFT **Many meridians end or begin in the hands.**

THE TWELVE REGULAR CHANNELS

The channels are generally named from their location rather than the organ they control. The solid organs (*Zang*) and Pericardium are associated with yin channels, while the hollow or *Fu* organs are matched with yang channels.

Affected organ	Meridian	Typical signs of disharmony
Lung	Hand *Tai Yin*	Coughs, asthma, chest pains
Large Intestine	Hand *Yang Ming*	Toothache, sore throats, neck pains
Spleen	Foot *Tai Yin*	Flatulence, vomiting, upper abdominal pain
Stomach	Foot *Yang Ming*	Abdominal bloating, vomiting, abdominal pain
Heart	Hand *Shao Yin*	Heart pain, palpitations, insomnia, night sweats
Small Intestine	Hand *Tai Yang*	Deafness, lower abdominal pain and distention
Kidney	Foot *Shao Yin*	Impotence, weakness in the lower limbs, increased frequency of urination
Urinary Bladder	Foot *Tai Yang*	Urinary retention, nasal catarrh, headache, back pain
Liver	Foot *Jue Yin*	Low back or abdominal pain, mental disturbances, hiccups
Gall Bladder	Foot *Shao Yang*	Headache, blurred vision, shoulder pain
Pericardium	Hand *Jue Yin*	Heart pain, poor concentration, palpitations
San Jiao	Hand *Shao Yang*	Abdominal bloating, deafness, tinnitus, urinary dysfunction

Each channel takes its name from the key organ it affects or, in the case of the extraordinary channels, its function. The number of acu points (*Xue Wei*) along the channels can vary significantly. These points are seen as sites where the *Qi* flowing through the channel is carried to the body's surface, so some sort of treatment at these sites – either with an acupuncture needle, applying pressure, or supplying heat in the form of moxabustion – will directly affect the flow of *Qi*.

In all, there are 361 regular points (on the main channels), of which around 150 are generally used by therapists. The number on each channel varies. The Heart meridian, for example, has only nine points, while the Urinary Bladder channel has the most with 67.

There are many more points, including the *Ah Shi* ("ah, yes") points, which are variable, tender and may appear only in particular diseases. There are also the "new points," discovered by therapists during practice. Ear acupuncture (*see* page 92) is almost a separate science, with about fifty points on the ear which relate to each organ of the body. In all, there are over 2,000 points.

THE EXTRAORDINARY CHANNELS

The eight extra channels include two regular or major channels: the "Governing Vessel" (*Du Mai*) and the "Conception Vessel" (*Ren Mai*).

The *Du Mai* governs all the yang channels and weakness here is associated with symptoms such as stiffness, back pain, and headaches. It runs from the anus, up the spine and across the crown of the head to finish inside the upper lip.

Ren also means "responsibility," and so the Conception Vessel is seen as being responsible for, or accountable to, all the other yin channels. It starts in the uterus and is particularly associated with pregnancy and childbirth. Miscarriage, for example, can be associated with weakness in the *Ren Mai*. General debility and physical weakness can also be linked to this channel.

The other six extra channels are:
• The "Penetrating Vessel" (*Chong Mai*), also called the "Sea of the twelve channels," since it communicates with the main channels. Like the *Ren Mai*, it starts from the uterus and can be associated with problems in pregnancy. Problems with this channel can also manifest as abdominal pains and muscle spasms.
• The "Girdle Vessel" (*Dai Mai*) runs around the waist like a belt and is usually described as "binding" all the channels together; problems here can be linked with back and abdominal pains.
• The *Yin Qiao*, or yin heel channel, runs along the inside of the heel, up the front of the body and ends near the eye. Excessive sleeping is regarded in terms of Chinese medicine as a symptom of disharmony in this channel.

• The *Yang Qiao*, or yang heel channel, starts on the outside of the heel and runs along the outer side of the leg and back to end at the back of the skull. Symptoms of disharmony here include insomnia and epilepsy.
• The *Yin Wei*, or yin tie channel, is so called, as it ties together the yin channels, connecting and regulating all of them. It starts at the front of the leg and ends in the neck. Heart pains can be a symptom of problems in this channel.
• The *Yang Wei*, or yang tie channel, fulfills a similar function to the *Yin Wei*, but only for the yang channels. It starts from the side of the foot and, like the *Yang Qiao*, ends at the back of the skull. Disharmony here may lead to such symptoms as chills and fevers.

As well as providing important links and connections for the twelve regular channels, these extra meridians also help to circulate *Jing* around the body and act as reservoirs for *Qi* and Blood, helping to keep the regular channels in balance.

The extra channels also play a part in circulating the *Wei Qi* (defense energy) around the body. Consequently, they are considered to be important in combating external evils and preventing disease.

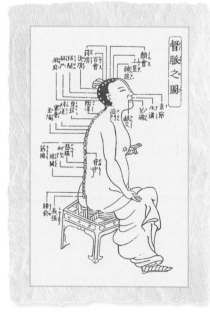

FAR LEFT *Ren Mai*, which governs the yin channel, and *Du Mai* (LEFT), which governs the yang channel, are two of the extraordinary channels. These channels act as reservoirs for *Qi* and Blood.

DAILY *QI* FLOW

Each day, our *Qi* travels through the network of channels in a well-defined rhythm. Any health problems with the associated organs are, therefore, most likely to manifest at a particular time each day – something which Western medicine would also support. The Lung channel, for example, is most dominant between 3 am and 5 am, so asthmatics often suffer severe symptoms in the early hours of the morning.

Regular sleep disturbances can suggest imbalance in a particular organ, but it is important to remember that these Chinese "organ concepts" do not exactly mirror Western ideas, so disharmony need not suggest a pathological problem, but may indicate an emotional or spiritual imbalance instead.

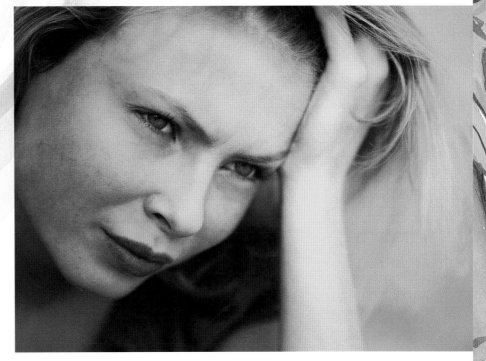

ABOVE **Regular sleep disturbances can suggest imbalance in a particular organ.**

DOMINANT MERIDIANS AND TIME OF DAY

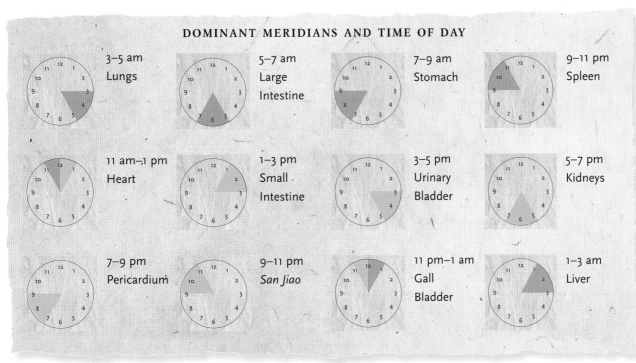

3–5 am
Lungs

5–7 am
Large
Intestine

7–9 am
Stomach

9–11 pm
Spleen

11 am–1 pm
Heart

1–3 pm
Small
Intestine

3–5 pm
Urinary
Bladder

5–7 pm
Kidneys

7–9 pm
Pericardium

9–11 pm
San Jiao

11 pm–1 am
Gall
Bladder

1–3 am
Liver

EXTERNAL CAUSES OF DISEASE

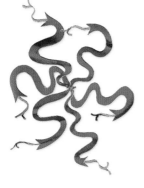

*T*he early Taoists regarded all disease simply as a sign of disharmony between yin and yang; however, Chinese physicians soon codified a complex set of possible causes of illness, focusing on both external and internal factors, including the six "evils."

SIX EVILS

Just as the ancient Greeks saw illness as a factor of changing climate, and early Europeans regarded it as caused by "flying venoms" that attacked the body, so Chinese tradition blames much ill health on similar external or exogenous factors.

The "six evils," commonly blamed for superficial illnesses, are best regarded – as in the Greek tradition – as changing environmental factors. In the central Asian steppes of ancient China, very hot, dry summers and cold winters are typical, with howling winds blowing regularly each spring.

So, not surprisingly, the key "evils" in Chinese medicine are:
• Wind
• Heat
• Summer Heat or Fire
• Cold
• Dryness
• Dampness.

Wind, Heat, Fire, and Dryness are all considered to be yang evils, while Cold and Damp are classified under this system as yin.

These evils each create characteristic symptoms – fevers and chills, for example, from Hot and Cold, or a shifting pattern of pain related to Wind. An attack of Dampness – characterized by symptoms like runny catarrh or edema – can develop into the more serious "Phlegm" regarded as an internal factor (*see* page 34), while Summer Heat is more commonly associated with tropical fevers than the chills of colder Northern climes.

A cold spring is regarded by Chinese physicians as a sure sign that there will be an excess of Cold-related disorders. Elderly Chinese people still persist in wearing hats or headscarves whenever out of doors to prevent an attack by Damp, which is traditionally regarded as especially likely to attack the head.

OTHER EXTERNAL EVILS

• Epidemic evils – the sort of serious infections and plagues that are now a rarity thanks to better public hygiene and heath care.
• Improper diet – regarded as a common cause of disease, since food is the source of much of our energy. Too much or too little food, irregular mealtimes, poor quality or polluted food will all lead to weakness and disharmony.
• Fatigue – which is seen as consuming *Qi*, and therefore weakens the body still further.

LEFT **The "six evils" (changing environmental factors causing illness) comprise yang evils Wind, Heat, Fire, and Dryness, and yin evils Cold and Damp.**

• Inactivity and too much leisure – the Chinese believe that inactivity will slow down the *Qi* and Blood circulation, leading to stagnation and dysfunction of Spleen and Stomach.

• Sexual indulgence – too much sex is seen as another external cause of ill health. Sexual activity is believed to deplete *Jing* and will lead to typical symptoms of Kidney deficiency, such as back pain and dizziness. The body is also believed to be especially prone to attack by the external evils during sexual intercourse, as the "body is open," so keeping warm and comfortable at this time is believed to be essential. Similarly, overfrequent childbirth is regarded as a possible cause of ill health in women, as it too will deplete the Kidney essence.

• Traumas and accidents also come into the "external causes" category,

and generally lead to direct damage to Blood or *Qi*.

• Insect and animal bites form the final category of exogenous disease factors – again, a problem that would be more significant in a semi-tropical world, where snakes and rabid dogs were commonplace, than in more sheltered environments.

External causes like these are regarded as more likely causes of illness in children or of "superficial" problems such as common colds or disorders like food poisoning which we now know to blame on bacteria or parasites. Adults are more likely to suffer from illness as a result of internal causes.

COMBINED ATTACK IN ARTHRITIS

The six evils can attack in combination: arthritis, for example, can be seen as a Cold, Damp, Wind problem in the shifting pattern of aches and twinges. Symptoms are usually worse when the weather is cold and wet. Arthritis, known as *Bi* syndrome in China (*Bi* = pain), can also be regarded as a Hot problem – the burning joints of rheumatoid arthritis, for example, would be a Hot, rather than Cold, condition.

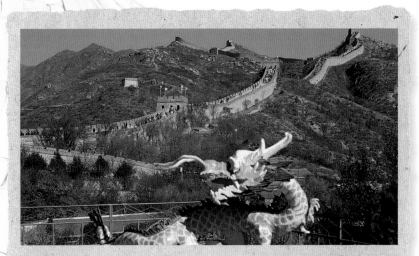

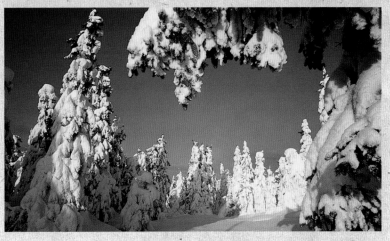

ABOVE **Summer Heat is more commonly associated with tropical fevers than the chills of colder Northern climes.**

33

INTERNAL CAUSES OF DISEASE

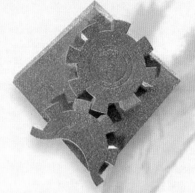

As well as external factors, Chinese medicine blames internal or endogenous factors for ill health. Some sicknesses are created by external evils, some by sufferers themselves. Both endogenous and external evils upset the body's balance and harmony.

THE SEVEN EMOTIONS

The seven emotions, which form an intrinsic part of the five-element model (*see* pages 20–21), are seen as the major internal cause of disease. An excess of any of them is likely to damage the organ connected with the emotion.

Too much worrying will damage the Spleen, and too much fear will affect the Kidney. In each case, the excess emotion interferes with the normal flow of *Qi*, with resulting symptoms and syndromes.

Too much anger, for example, will cause the Liver *Qi* to rise, resulting in headache, facial flushing, and ultimately – in severe cases – an increased risk of a stroke. Treatment involves using herbs or acupuncture to help reverse this upward Liver *Qi* flow, as well as encouraging the patient to take a calmer view of the world.

PHLEGM

The Chinese view of Phlegm goes rather beyond the Western concept of it as a sort of catarrhal mucus produced during vigorous bouts of coughing. There are believed to be two sorts of Phlegm – visible and invisible.

The visible is our familiar sputum, but the invisible collects inside the body and can be both a product and cause of disease. Spleen *Qi* deficiency, for example, will lead to production of Phlegm, which will then move toward the Heart and cause a blockage. This is seen as a cause of mental disorders such as schizophrenia, since the Heart is the key focus for mental activity.

Phlegm production is closely associated with the Spleen's role in separating the clear and turbid fluids produced during digestion. Phlegm tends to be stored by the Lungs –

hence its physical manifestation in productive coughing.

Asthma is also associated with excess Phlegm. Its characteristic wheeziness is described as the "sound of Phlegm."

Typical symptoms of Phlegm syndrome include a thick, greasy coating to the tongue and a slippery or wiry pulse (*see* pages 40–43). Other symptoms will depend on where the Phlegm is concentrated. If it is in the stomach, it will lead to nausea and vomiting; if in the Lungs, to coughing and shortness of breath; in the Heart, to mental disturbances, coma, delirium, and so on.

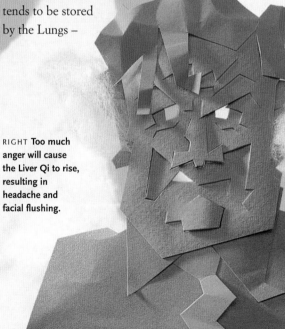

RIGHT **Too much anger will cause the Liver Qi to rise, resulting in headache and facial flushing.**

BLOOD STASIS

The third important cause of internal illness is Blood stasis or stagnation. Again, one must recall that "Blood" in the Chinese context means rather more than the Western anatomical concept of the red stuff circulating in our veins and arteries. Blood stasis, like invisible Phlegm, is seen as some sort of blockage in the normal circulation – but that doesn't always mean the Western concept of a blood clot or thrombosis.

Blood stasis can be caused by a number of factors, including:
• *Qi* stagnation
• *Qi* deficiency
• Cold entering the Blood, causing it to congeal and slow down

• Heat entering the Blood, increasing the flow and leading to hemorrhage, and
• traumatic injuries or wounds.

Blood stasis is often associated with a stabbing pain, enlargement or swelling of the body organs, purplish spots on the tongue (*see* page 40), or some sort of bleeding.

CONGENITAL PROBLEMS

We can do very little about some internal causes of disease factors – fetal damage or inherent birth defects are both in this category – but that doesn't prevent parents from trying.

In Southern China, it is still common to give new-born babies a herbal brew at fifteen days of age designed to clear the heat and toxins that are believed to be present at birth.

Premature birth is seen as a potential cause of internal illness. The mother's health during pregnancy also is significant and can have a fundamental influence on the subsequent vigor and vitality of her offspring.

The "congenital *Qi*" (*see* page 24) that we are born with is something that it is very difficult for us to do much about.

BELOW **A normal birth and healthy baby are important factors for long-term health. Congenital weakness is often blamed for chronic illness.**

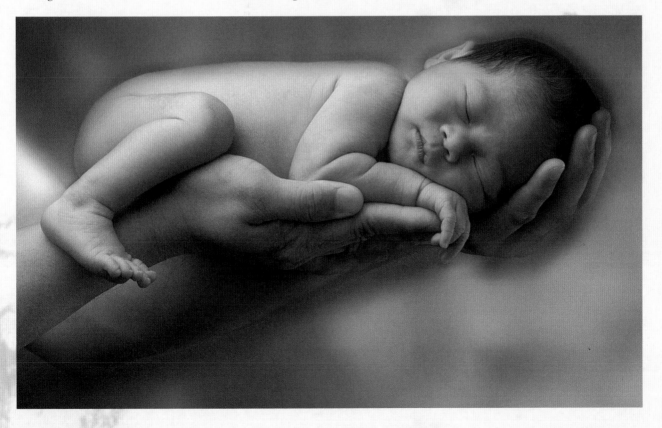

CHINESE PATHOLOGY

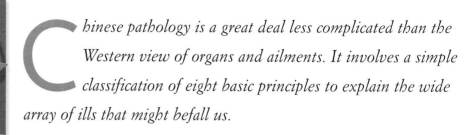

*C*hinese pathology is a great deal less complicated than the Western view of organs and ailments. It involves a simple classification of eight basic principles to explain the wide array of ills that might befall us.

DIFFERENTIATING SYNDROMES

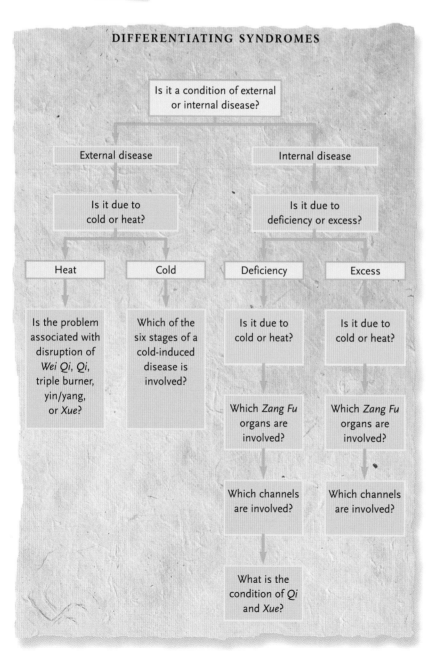

Is it a condition of external or internal disease?

External disease

Internal disease

Is it due to cold or heat?

Is it due to deficiency or excess?

Heat

Cold

Deficiency

Excess

Is the problem associated with disruption of *Wei Qi, Qi,* triple burner, yin/yang, or *Xue?*

Which of the six stages of a cold-induced disease is involved?

Is it due to cold or heat?

Is it due to cold or heat?

Which *Zang Fu* organs are involved?

Which *Zang Fu* organs are involved?

Which channels are involved?

Which channels are involved?

What is the condition of *Qi* and *Xue?*

THE EIGHT GUIDING PRINCIPLES

For the Chinese, illness is not a matter of invading microorganisms, diseased or damaged tissues, or stress-related problems. It can involve four simple possibilities:

• the division into interior or exterior causes of disease (*see* pages 32–34)

• a basic confrontation between the body's vital energy and an invading evil

• imbalances in yin and yang, or

• a problem with *Qi* circulation.

These factors form the basis of all Chinese disease syndromes and are sometimes summarized as the eight principles, or *Ba Gang*, involving:

Deficiency	Excess
Cold	Heat
Yin	Yang
Interior	Exterior

Diagnosis is simply a matter of logically considering these possibilities and identifying the underlying cause of the problem.

LEFT **The Chinese physician differentiates syndromes through a structured series of examinations and questions.**

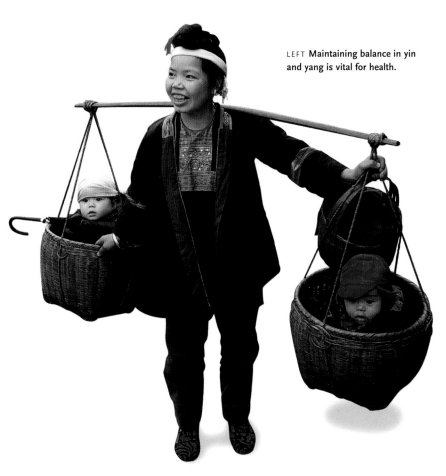

LEFT **Maintaining balance in yin and yang is vital for health.**

MEETING EVILS

If the *Qi* is strong and the evil is weak, then there are no problems. If the *Qi* is weak and the evils stronger, that is a different matter.

Chinese pathology sees three distinct outcomes:
• If the *Qi* is strong and the evil is also strong, then the result is an Excess Syndrome.
• If the *Qi* is weak and the evil is also weak, then the result is a Deficiency Syndrome.
• If the *Qi* is weak and the evil is strong, the result will be a mixed Excess and Deficiency Syndrome.

IMBALANCE IN YIN AND YANG

Yin and yang are present in all things. They balance and complement each other and cannot exist in isolation. However, if yin and yang get out of balance, with one becoming too weak or too strong, then the scene is set for illness. As with the *Qi* versus evil confrontation, a number of options will determine the disease syndrome:
• If yin is too strong and yang is normal, the result is a Cold Syndrome.
• If yin is normal and yang is too strong, the result is a Heat Syndrome.
• If yin is strong and yang is weak, then the result is a Cold Deficiency Syndrome.
• If yin is weak and yang is strong, then the result is a Hot Deficiency Syndrome.

PROBLEMS WITH *QI* CIRCULATION

Different types of *Qi* (*see* pages 24–25) circulate around the body in different ways. Lung *Qi*, for example, normally rises while the Lungs are also involved in the body's water circulation, ensuring that fluids go downward. If, instead, the Lung *Qi* goes down, then the water flow is also interrupted and rises instead, and the result can be coughing and edema.

Similarly, Spleen *Qi* rises, but if it falls instead, then there is insufficient energy going to the head, so the person starts to feel dizzy. Stomach *Qi* is heavier and so falls, but if it does not, then it stays in the abdomen, creating a sensation of fullness and bloating, possibly leading to constipation.

Interfering with the normal *Qi* circulation associated with each of the body's organs leads to an equivalent set of symptoms, which the Chinese physician uses to identify exactly where the problem lies. Imbalance in the *Qi* circulation, in turn, affects the fine relationship between yin and yang – tipping the seesaw one way or another and adding to the resulting syndrome.

> 66 If yin and yang separate, one's essence and vital force will be destroyed. If then the evening dew and the wind touch one, they will cause chills and fever. This is how one is hurt by the wind, and then the evil influences will remain in the body and create a leakage. 99
>
> *HUANG DI NEI JING*

CHINESE DIAGNOSTICS

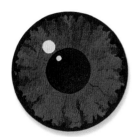

*U*nlike today's doctors, early Chinese physicians could only depend on their own observation skills for diagnosis. No invasive tests or complex monitoring systems were available, just the basic techniques of looking, listening, and touching.

SKILLED OBSERVATION

Accurate diagnosis in traditional Chinese medicine depends entirely on the physician's observational skills. A good doctor can pull together an array of inferences in the patient's physical appearance, pulse, voice, or demeanor to pinpoint the relevant syndrome.

The Chinese divide diagnostics into four distinct methods or techniques:
• Inspection or looking – the most important component – which involves examining the patient's appearance, tongue, nose, skin color, and so on.
• Auscultation and olfaction – hearing and smelling – which includes listening to the patient's voice and breathing rhythms, and smelling any body odors. In the past, "taste" was added to this stage in the diagnosis, and physicians would regularly taste their patients' urine to identify any sweetness which could imply diabetes.
• Interrogation – the "asking questions" stage identifying how the patient feels – hot, cold, thirsty, hungry, or in pain.
• Palpation or touching – this includes the complexities of Chinese pulse taking, as well as feeling the body surface to assess temperature and quality, and check for any swellings.

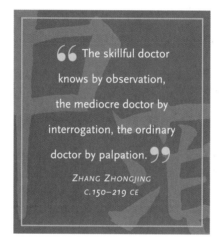

66 The skillful doctor knows by observation, the mediocre doctor by interrogation, the ordinary doctor by palpation. 99

ZHANG ZHONGJING
C.150–219 CE

BELOW **Different parts of the eye indicate to the skilled physician the health and strength of the five *Zang* organs.**

INSPECTION

Accurate inspection is the most important of the Chinese doctor's diagnostic skills, and goes very far beyond the sort of cursory glance that most Western physicians bestow on their patients. Although the list of points to inspect is long, the skilled practitioner will see and identify these various characteristics comparatively quickly.

The process starts with a "general inspection," looking not just at the patient's build and posture but identifying the "body spirit" – whether the patient seems bright and

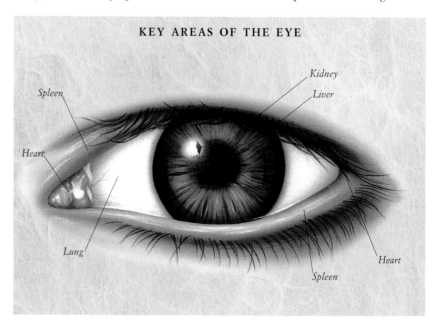

KEY AREAS OF THE EYE

Spleen
Kidney
Liver
Heart
Lung
Heart
Spleen

alert, or downcast and withdrawn. This spirit is believed by Chinese physicians to be best seen in the eyes, sometimes called the "door of the spirit," and the practitioner will look to see whether the indivdual's eyes are bright and shiny, as well as noting any characteristic coloration in the sclera (white of the eye) or eyelids, and if the eyes are alert and responsive.

The area around the eye is believed to indicate the quality of the main body organs. Swollen eyelids, for example, might well suggest Spleen deficiency, while yellowish discharges in the corners of the eyes would suggest some sort of Heat problem with the Heart.

Bright eyes suggest a strong and full spirit, but if they have a shiny/glassy appearance it means that the spirit is weak (sometimes termed "false spirit"). Red eyes usually indicate a Heat problem, while, if the sclera is yellow in appearance, it implies a Damp problem.

The color of the face is also important, while the shape of the body suggests the quality of *Qi* and *Jing*:
• a firm, muscular body suggests that *Qi* and *Jing* are strong and the person is intrinsically healthy
• obesity and fat can imply Spleen *Qi* deficiency or an excess of Phlegm and Dampness
• a thin body with poor appetite implies some sort of digestive weakness – typically Middle *Jiao* deficiency

• on the other hand, a thin body with a good appetite is likely to suggest yin deficiency or overactivity in the Middle *Jiao*.

Inspection also involves observing the patient's behavior and movements – someone who is overactive and always moving might be suffering from a yang syndrome or some problem of excess of Heat, while a more static individual inclined to sit and do nothing is more likely to be suffering from a Cold or deficiency syndrome or an imbalance affecting yin.

Any tremors are also carefully noted – in the elderly, shaking hands imply yin deficiency, while in younger people it is more likely to be related to a Wind problem.

The inspection process also includes detailed examination of different parts of the body – the head hair, for example, is closely linked with the Kidneys in the five-element model, so its quality can give some indication of underlying Kidney energies. Thinning or graying hair can suggest Kidney *Qi* or *Jing* deficiency, while hair loss and baldness can imply Blood deficiency or a problem with Wind invading the head. Greasy, oily hair usually suggests some sort of Damp syndrome.

The strength of the *Du Mai* (the governing channel) is also indicated by the condition of the head. An unusually small head, for example, suggests an inherent weakness in the channels and chronic health problems.

FACIAL COLORS AND LIKELY ASSOCIATED SYNDROMES

Red	Heat syndrome
Flushed red	Excessive heat
Malar flush *(across the cheekbones) or flushing only in the evenings*	Yin or Heat deficiency
Yellow	Dampness, or Spleen or Blood deficiency
Dull yellow	Cold and Damp syndrome
Clear yellow	Heat and Damp syndrome
White	Cold syndrome
Pale	*Qi* or yang deficiency
Green	Cold syndrome, or possibly pain or Blood stagnation
Black	Cold syndrome, or possibly pain or yang deficiency

TONGUE INSPECTION

The tongue is very indicative of disease. Chinese medical textbooks always include dozens of illustrations of characteristic tongue shapes and colors for the medical student to study and learn.

As with the eyes, the various parts of the tongue are believed to relate to particular body organs. It is sometimes called the "map of the body." So the physician will take careful note of where any swellings or blemishes actually occur.

Just as with the face, the various colors that can be seen in the tongue suggest particular syndromes. The shape and size of the tongue is also important. A swollen tongue can suggest excess heat in the Heart or Spleen, for example, while a thin, pale tongue would indicate deficiency of *Qi* and Blood.

Cracks in the tongue or toothmarks at the edges provide the physician with additional clues about the underlying syndrome. A pale, cracked appearance, for example, would suggest a Blood deficiency, while toothmarks at the edges would imply a Spleen yang deficiency.

The coating of the tongue is also important in diagnostic terms. This should normally be thin, moist and white. If it has a yellow tinge, the doctor will suspect a Heat syndrome or an internal health problem; if thick and white, it implies the patient is suffering from a superficial syndrome or a Cold problem.

There are dozens of possible combinations involving tongue color, coating, shape, blemishes, and motion. Each will suggest a specific syndrome or health problem to the experienced practitioner.

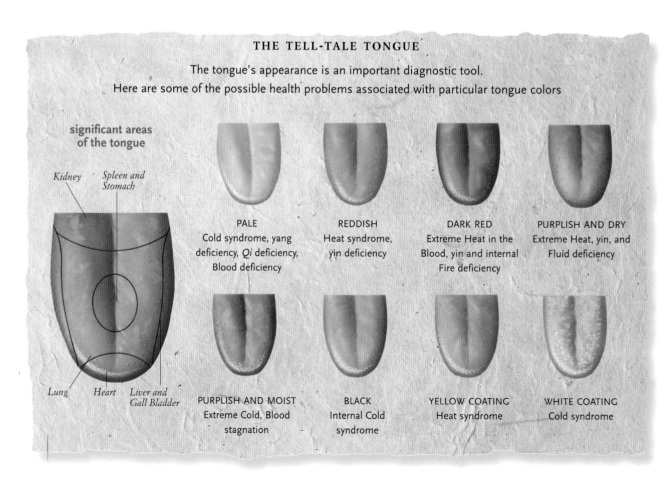

THE TELL-TALE TONGUE

The tongue's appearance is an important diagnostic tool.
Here are some of the possible health problems associated with particular tongue colors

significant areas of the tongue

Kidney

Spleen and Stomach

Lung

Heart

Liver and Gall Bladder

PALE
Cold syndrome, yang deficiency, *Qi* deficiency, Blood deficiency

REDDISH
Heat syndrome, yin deficiency

DARK RED
Extreme Heat in the Blood, yin and internal Fire deficiency

PURPLISH AND DRY
Extreme Heat, yin, and Fluid deficiency

PURPLISH AND MOIST
Extreme Cold, Blood stagnation

BLACK
Internal Cold syndrome

YELLOW COATING
Heat syndrome

WHITE COATING
Cold syndrome

READING THE NOSE

Various points on the nose are considered by practitioners to correspond to different parts of the body and are similarly used in diagnosis by noting the color or quality of each area. For example, spots around the end of the nose would suggest a Stomach or Spleen Heat problem.

On the other hand, since the nose is controlled by the Lung, any nasal blemishes would be considered as possibly indicating an underlying Lung problem.

AUSCULTATION AND OLFACTION

Having completed a thorough inspection, the physician will move on to the "listening and smelling" part of the process. If the patient has a loud voice, the problem is more likely to be one of Heat or Excess, while a soft voice implies Cold or Deficiency. Speech is associated with the Heart, so any discontinuities or speech impediments can suggest a problem with the physical heart, the circulation, or mental activities, which the Chinese also link to the Heart.

The physician will also pay particular attention to the patient's breath. If it is fast, then it may suggest Heat in the Lungs. If it is shallow, there may be a problem with Kidney *Qi* deficiency.

Coughing is associated with rising Lung *Qi*, while hiccups imply ascending Stomach *Qi*.

The physician will be busy smelling the patient too. Strong body odor generally suggests a Heat problem. For example, bad breath would seem to suggest Heat in the Stomach.

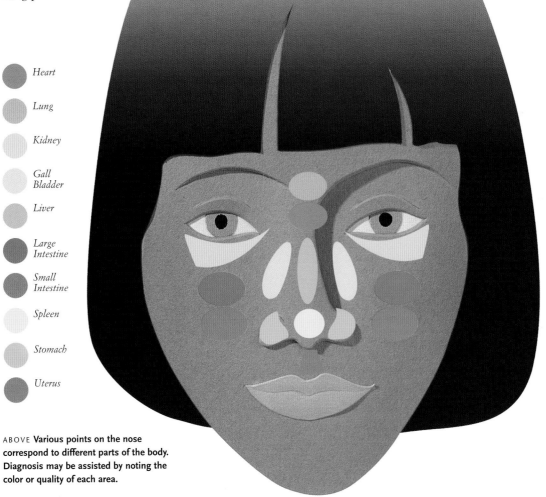

Heart

Lung

Kidney

Gall Bladder

Liver

Large Intestine

Small Intestine

Spleen

Stomach

Uterus

ABOVE **Various points on the nose correspond to different parts of the body. Diagnosis may be assisted by noting the color or quality of each area.**

41

INTERROGATION

Interrogation to the Chinese physician is less about taking a conventional Western-style case history, than asking the patient how he or she "feels" – whether they feel hot or cold, are thirsty or hungry, have a tendency to sweat or shiver, or feel a need to keep warm.

The doctor will also ask about pain, not just whether there is any, but the exact quality of the pain, that is, whether it is heavy, gnawing, hot, cold, spasmodic etc. Western patients find it difficult to describe the quality of the pain they feel, but the Chinese are very familiar with the doctors' classification system and will provide graphic details of the exact nature of any pains to help with the diagnosis.

The patient will also be asked about bowel motions, sleeping patterns, urination, and – if women – menstruation. While a Western practitioner may be interested simply in how much or when, the Chinese physician will be looking for precise information. When exactly does the patient wake at night? What particular sorts of food does he or she crave or avoid? What is the exact appearance of menstrual blood?

This degree of detail may seem strange to Westerners, but it is essential if the Chinese doctor is to pinpoint the exact syndrome and underlying imbalances.

PALPATION

The final stage of the diagnosis is usually touching – feeling the body to assess temperature and the nature of any swellings, as in Western medicine, but also taking very careful note of the pulse.

While Western medicine regards the pulses – at wrist, neck, foot or wherever – as simply indicating heartbeat, Chinese medicine focuses on subtle variations in the quality and texture of the pulse.

The key position is the wrists (radial pulse) where the Chinese doctor will actually feel nine different and individual pulses.

The doctor's three middle fingers are used, each corresponding to a slightly different position on the wrist which represents a particular body organ.

In addition, the physician will slightly vary the pressure he or she applies to each wrist to feel the nature of the pulse at three different levels – on the surface of the wrist (superficial), with a little pressure

LEFT **Interrogation is an important part of the consultation, with the physician looking for the numerous minute changes in symptoms, moods or dislikes that will indicate the underlying syndrome.**

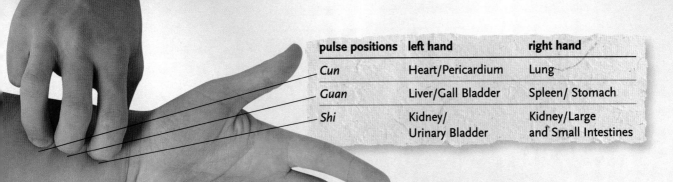

pulse positions	left hand	right hand
Cun	Heart/Pericardium	Lung
Guan	Liver/Gall Bladder	Spleen/ Stomach
Shi	Kidney/ Urinary Bladder	Kidney/Large and Small Intestines

applied (middle), and finally pressing quite hard against the patient's wrist (deep).

The practitioner also measures the pulse rate – not by counting against a clock as in the West, but by timing the pulse to his own steady breathing, with four pulses per breath (at a rate of around eighteen breaths per minute) deemed to be normal. More important than the rate is the actual quality of each pulse. A healthy, normal pulse is strong without being "solid," with a regular rhythm and a firm root – felt by pressing deeply in the *Shi* position.

The quality of the pulse will vary through the year:
• in the spring, it is described as slightly "wiry"
• in summer, "full"
• in late summer, "softer"
• in the fall, it is slightly "floating"
• in the winter, it is more likely to be "deep."

These textures mirror the quality of the seasons in the five-element model. Wiry, for example, corresponds to the Liver, spring, and Wood.

Many of these terms are difficult to appreciate without actually being able to feel what a "wiry" pulse is, and what is "floating." Skilled pulse diagnosis is a precise art which can take years to perfect.

ABNORMAL PULSES AND THEIR INDICATIONS

Type	Syndrome
Floating	Superficial syndromes, e.g., colds
Deep	Internal syndromes
Slow	Cold syndrome; yang deficiency
Rapid	Heat syndrome
Weak	Deficiency syndromes
Solid/hard	Excess syndromes
Smooth/slippery	Phlegm/Damp syndromes; usual pulse in pregnancy
Rough	*Qi* or Blood stagnation; Blood or *Jing* deficiency
Thready/feeble	*Qi* and Blood deficiency; Damp syndromes
Full	Heat excess
Wiry	Liver or Gall Bladder imbalance/pain; Phlegm or Damp syndromes
Irregular – slow/weak	*Qi* exhaustion; *Qi* and Blood deficiency; yang deficiency
Irregular – slow/breaking	Cold or Phlegm stagnation; Blood stagnation
Irregular – rapid/breaking	Heat excess; *Qi* or Blood stagnation; Phlegm syndromes
Very deep/hidden	Extreme pain; yang *Qi* exhaustion
Very fast	Extreme yang excess; yin exhaustion
Very weak	*Qi* and Blood deficiency; yang exhaustion
Long (beyond *Shi* position)	Excess syndromes; Heat syndrome; *Qi* stagnation
Short (no *Guan* or *Shi*)	*Qi* deficiency; *Qi* depression

TREATING EXTERIOR SYNDROMES

*U*sing the eight guiding principles and traditional diagnostic techniques, the Chinese physician aims to identify the exact syndrome complex from which the patient suffers – syndromes often sound very different from the familiar disorders of Western medicine.

SUPERFICIAL PROBLEMS

Into the "exterior syndromes" category fall the sorts of diseases which in Western medicine we would blame on colds and infections: the sort of self-limiting ailments that start suddenly, flare up, and just as quickly subside.

To identify them, the Chinese practitioner asks detailed questions about how the problem started, whether the patient feels hot or cold, and whether the person is suffering from a headache, coughing or catarrh. The tongue and pulse are examined.

Exterior syndromes are generally related directly to attack by the six external evils – wind, heat, cold, fire, dampness, and dryness – usually in combination. The result is a complex list of possible exterior syndromes: Wind–Cold, Wind–Heat, and Summer Heat are just three of them.

WIND–COLD IN THE EXTERIOR

This is characterized by an aversion to cold, slight fever, headache, aches and pains in the limbs, a thin white coating to the tongue, and a floating, tight pulse. Wind is usually associated with movement, so the practitioner would be interested in whether the aches and pains shifted around the body or were always located in one particular place. Equivalent Western ailments could include chills, the common cold, or influenza.

A suitable Chinese herbal remedy would use warming, pungent herbs to encourage sweating. Many of the herbs traditionally used for this are also antimicrobials to help combat infection.

A typical Chinese formula for Wind and Cold attacking the exterior would be *Gui Zhi Tang* (cinnamon twig decoction), which is made from *Gui Zhi* (6g), *Bai Shao* (6g), *Sheng Jiang* (3g), *Gan Cao* (3g), and *Da Zao* (3g). This is diaphoretic and strengthening for the *Wei Qi* (*see* pages 58–81 for full details of these herbs).

In addition, a Chinese physician might use acupuncture: LI20 (*Yingxiang*) for clearing nasal catarrh or *Taiyang* for a headache (*see* pages 88–93 and pages 114–129 for details of these points).

BELOW **Many herbs are used in treating illnesses related to external problems.**

Rou Dou Kou (nutmeg)

Chuan Xiong (Sichuan lovage)

Bai Shao (white peony)

Chi Shao (red peony)

WIND–HEAT IN THE EXTERIOR

This is characterized by a fever, slight intolerance to wind and cold, headache, red eyes, thick nasal catarrh, sore throat, redness on the sides and tip of the tongue, thirst, yellow urine, and a floating, rapid pulse. There may also be a rash or skin eruption developing.

These sorts of symptoms would be associated in the West with feverish colds, or perhaps a cold which started as a chill (Cold in the exterior), which becomes more severe as the infection takes hold. It might also indicate the early stages of measles, chicken pox or tonsillitis.

A typical remedy for Wind–Heat would be *Yin Qiao San* (honeysuckle and forsythia powder), which is a complex remedy of ten herbs. The most important are *Jin Yin Hua* (9g), *Lian Qiao* (9g), *Niu Bang Zi* (6g), *Bo He* (3g), and *Jie Geng* (6g). Several of these herbs are strongly antimicrobial, or, as the Chinese would say, they "dispel fire poisons."

For the sore throat, a practitioner might also use acupuncture – perhaps at LU11 (*Shaoshang*).

*Bo He
(field mint)*

*Xuan Shen
(ningpo figwort)*

ATTACK BY SUMMER HEAT (FIRE)

Typical symptoms would include fever, excessive sweating, restlessness, a general lack of energy or lassitude, and a marked thirst for cold drinks. This is the sort of problem that would be described in the West as a "summer cold." This could develop with dizziness and nausea to what Westerners would describe as heatstroke or sunstroke.

In subtropical southern China, Summer Heat is commonly associated with dampness, where the sufferer feels even less energetic, with a poor appetite and probably diarrhea.

Traditional remedies for Summer Heat include cooling and energy-giving herbs, as well as antimicrobials. Typical is *Qing Shu Yi Qi Tang* (decoction to clear summer heat and replenish *Qi*), another complex formula of fifteen herbs, including: *Huang Qi* (9g), *Dang Gui* (6g), *Ze Xie* (6g), *Mai Men Dong* (6g), *Bai Zhu* (3g), *Cang Zhu* (3g), *Qing Pi* (3g), *Wu Wei Zi* (3g), and *Ren Shen* (1g).

Acupuncture at ST36 (*Zusanli*) might be added to the treatment to help stimulate the appetite.

BELOW **After identifying whether the syndrome's cause is external or internal, the physician can further classify it following the eight principles.**

DIAGNOSING EXTERIOR CONDITIONS

EXTERNAL DISEASE

Is it due to cold or heat?

Heat

Cold

Is the problem associated with disruption of *Wei Qi*, *Qi*, triple burner, yin/yang, or *Xue*?

Which of the six stages of a cold-induced disease is involved?

TREATING INTERIOR SYNDROMES

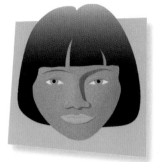

nterior syndromes are considered to be more serious than the superficial and self-limiting external ailments and can often be related to specific organ problems as well as energy imbalances.

IDENTIFYING THE PROBLEM

While exterior syndromes are mainly equated with chills or infections, the "interior syndromes" category covers virtually everything else – from major heart problems such as angina pectoris and coronary heart disease to menopausal upsets or period pain. Again, the eight guiding principles and traditional diagnostic methods are applied in a logical pattern to pinpoint where the imbalances might occur, or which of the *Zang Fu* organs may be affected.

Chinese medicine argues that there are three ways for an interior syndrome to develop:

• An exterior condition which has not been treated in time or adequately might be transmitted to the interior.

• The internal organs might be invaded directly by the external pathogens – such as Interior Cold caused by eating too much cold or raw food.

• The organs may be affected by emotional disturbances, which may lead to deficient functionality.

There are an enormous number of interior syndromes, each with a characteristic set of symptoms that can be difficult to translate neatly into a conventional Western disease label.

LUNG INVASION

Among the "excess" problems that might affect the Lung would be invasion by Wind–Cold. This could be a progression from the common cold that an attacking evil would cause in the exterior (*see* pages 44–45). The symptoms would be very similar, but there may also be watery nasal catarrh and a cough with white, mucus-like sputum. In the West, this might be labeled as a chest infection or simply a bad cold. A typical prescription for this sort of condition would be *Xing Su San* (apricot seed and perilla powder), which has around eleven herbs, including *Xing Ren* (6g), *Zi Su Ye* (6g), *Zhi Ke* (6g), *Jie Geng* (6g), *Ban Xia* (6g), *Fu Ling* (9g), and *Sheng Jiang* (3g). Like *Gui Zhi Tang*, this is a warming, diaphoretic mixture, with the addition of herbs like *Zhi Ke* to help to reverse the flow of *Qi*, which is blamed for sputum and coughs.

Xing Ren (bitter apricot)

Wind–Heat invading the Lungs, another excess condition, would be characterized by the same symptoms as Wind–Heat in the exterior, but with an additional cough and thick yellow sputum. In the West this might be labeled as acute bronchitis. A typical Chinese herbal remedy would be *Sang Ju Yin* (decoction of mulberry leaf and chrysanthemum), which includes among its main ingredients *Sang Ye* (6g), *Ju Hua* (3g), *Xing Ren* (6g) and *Jie Geng* (6g), as well as the *Bo He* and *Lian Qiao* from Yin Qiao San. If the sputum was profuse then the physician might add *Zhe Bei Mu* to the mix as well.

A Chinese practitioner might advise cupping across the chest area to relieve any pain.

Zi Su Ye (purple perill

Sheng Jiang (ginger)

Sang Ye (mulberry)

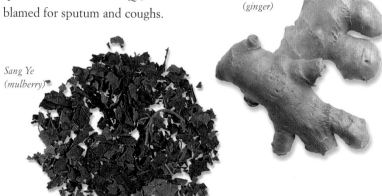

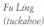
Fu Ling
(tuckahoe)

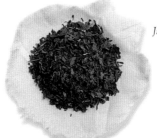
Ju Hua (chrysanthemum)

EXCESSIVE SADNESS

The emotions associated with the Lungs are grief and sadness, and these may be the cause of similar cough-like symptoms, as excess emotions weaken the Lungs and lead to *Qi* deficiency. This can be a cause of bronchitis or asthmatic conditions, and it is not that unusual for a bereavement (friend, family, or even a pet animal) to trigger this sort of syndrome.

Typical symptoms would include shortness of breath, cough or wheeziness, copious thin sputum, lassitude and tiredness, a weak or feeble-sounding voice, a pale or dry tongue with white coating, an empty and weak pulse. One of the most effective herbs for this sort of Lung *Qi* deficiency is *Ren Shen*, used alone, or a physician might feel that *Shen Mai San* (activate vascular system powder) could be a suitable remedy. This contains 6–9g each of *Ren Shen*, *Mai Men Dong*, and *Wu Wei Zi*.

Acupuncture at PC6 (*Neiguan*) or RM17 (*Shanzhong*) might be used for any chest pain.

Jie Geng (balloon flower)

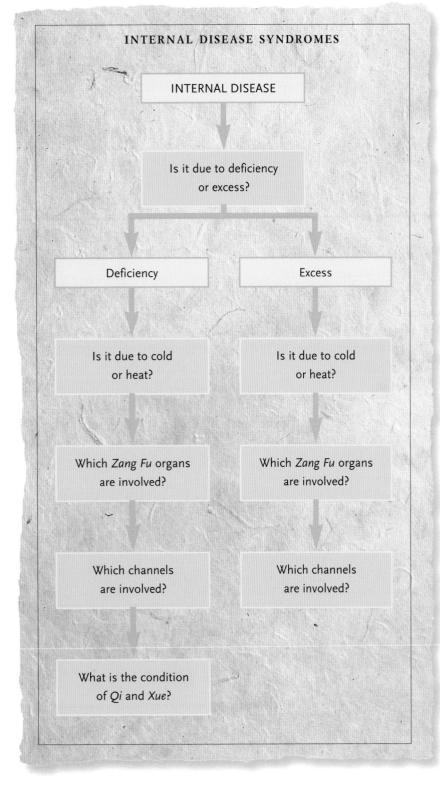

INTERNAL DISEASE SYNDROMES

INTERNAL DISEASE

Is it due to deficiency or excess?

Deficiency

Excess

Is it due to cold or heat?

Is it due to cold or heat?

Which *Zang Fu* organs are involved?

Which *Zang Fu* organs are involved?

Which channels are involved?

Which channels are involved?

What is the condition of *Qi* and *Xue*?

FINDING THE SYNDROME

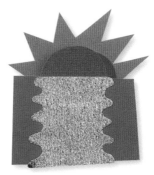

Interpreting *Western ailments in Chinese terms finds a variety of causes to blame that are generally unfamiliar to the Western way of thinking about health and illness. Energy imbalances, dampness, stagnation, and fundamental weaknesses are the main culprits in producing illness.*

LOW BACK PAIN

In Western medicine, low back pain is variously blamed on urinary tract disorders, rheumatism, spinal problems, or muscle strains. In Chinese theory, the nearby Kidneys are considered more likely to be involved and the possible causes of low back pain are:

• Damp–Cold in the lumbar region interrupting *Qi* and Blood flows, typically caused by lying on cold, damp ground

• Damp–Heat obstructing the channels

• excessive consumption of Kidney *Jing*, possibly associated with old age or too much sexual activity, or

• stagnation of *Qi* and Blood as a result of traumatic injuries or chronic illness.

Differentiation factors for the physician include whether the patient feels cold or hot, the nature of the tongue coating – slimy white for Damp–Cold problems, slimy yellow for Damp–Heat (associated symptoms like tinnitus and dizziness, which would imply Kidney weakness), or a dark red tongue and a fixed, stinging pain which would suggest Blood stagnation.

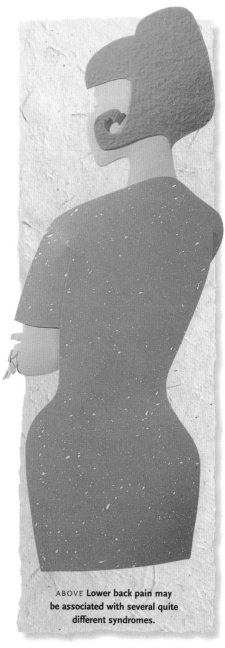

ABOVE **Lower back pain may be associated with several quite different syndromes.**

Once the syndrome has been exactly classified, then the relevant herbal formula can be chosen. Back pain associated with Kidney weakness, for example, might be treated with *Qing E Wan* (translated in some texts rather delightfully as "The blue fairy lady pills for lumbago").

This contains equal amounts of *Bu Gu Zhi, Du Zhong, Hu Tao Ren,* and *Da Suan* – taken in 9g doses twice a day. These herbs all help to encourage Kidney energy.

Moxabustion at DM4 (*Mingmen*) might also be used to help stimulate the Kidneys.

If excess Cold and Dampness after sitting in wet grass is at fault, then a remedy like *Du Huo Ji Sheng Tang* (angelica and mistletoe decoction) might be more suitable. This contains fifteen herbs, including *Du Huo* (6g), *Fang Feng* (3g), *Sang Ji Sheng* (6g), *Du Zhong* (3g), *Niu Xi* (3g), *Rou Gui* (1g), *Dang Gui* (3g), *Chuan Xiong* (3g), *Shu Di Huang* (3g), *Bai Shao* (3g), *Ren Shen* (3g), *Fu Ling* (9g), and *Gan Cao* (3g), and will help to warm the Kidneys and Liver, as well as clearing Cold and Damp.

Acupuncture at UB23 (*Shenshu*) and UB40 (*Weizhong*) might also be included in the treatment.

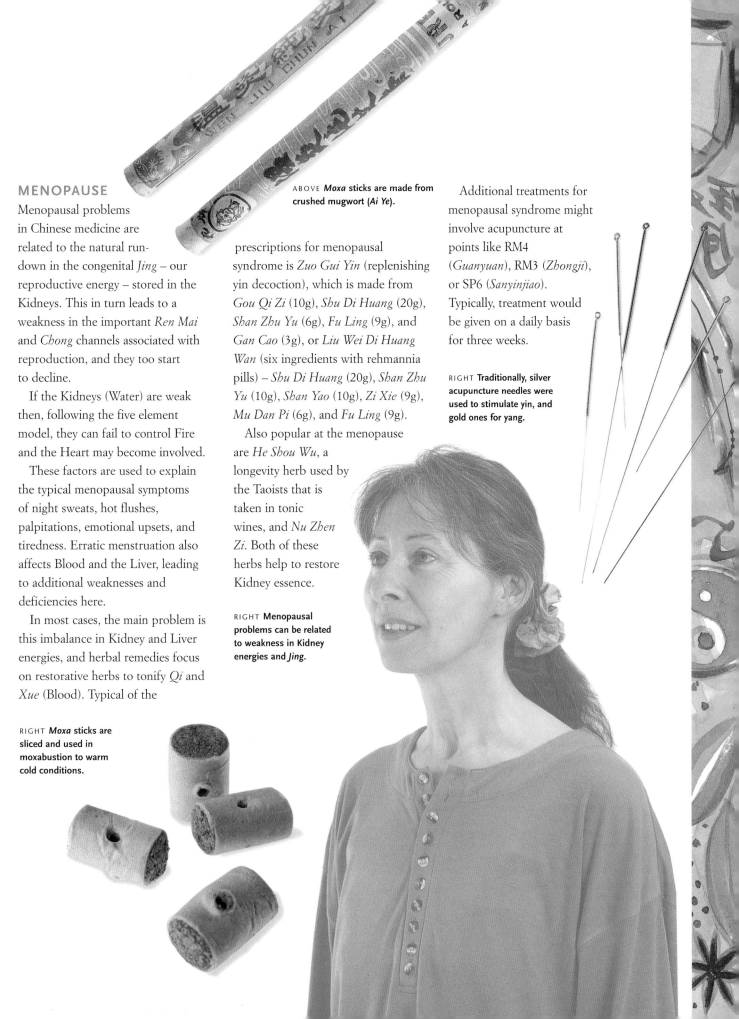

ABOVE **Moxa** sticks are made from crushed mugwort (**Ai Ye**).

MENOPAUSE

Menopausal problems in Chinese medicine are related to the natural run-down in the congenital *Jing* – our reproductive energy – stored in the Kidneys. This in turn leads to a weakness in the important *Ren Mai* and *Chong* channels associated with reproduction, and they too start to decline.

If the Kidneys (Water) are weak then, following the five element model, they can fail to control Fire and the Heart may become involved.

These factors are used to explain the typical menopausal symptoms of night sweats, hot flushes, palpitations, emotional upsets, and tiredness. Erratic menstruation also affects Blood and the Liver, leading to additional weaknesses and deficiencies here.

In most cases, the main problem is this imbalance in Kidney and Liver energies, and herbal remedies focus on restorative herbs to tonify *Qi* and *Xue* (Blood). Typical of the

prescriptions for menopausal syndrome is *Zuo Gui Yin* (replenishing yin decoction), which is made from *Gou Qi Zi* (10g), *Shu Di Huang* (20g), *Shan Zhu Yu* (6g), *Fu Ling* (9g), and *Gan Cao* (3g), or *Liu Wei Di Huang Wan* (six ingredients with rehmannia pills) – *Shu Di Huang* (20g), *Shan Zhu Yu* (10g), *Shan Yao* (10g), *Zi Xie* (9g), *Mu Dan Pi* (6g), and *Fu Ling* (9g).

Also popular at the menopause are *He Shou Wu*, a longevity herb used by the Taoists that is taken in tonic wines, and *Nu Zhen Zi*. Both of these herbs help to restore Kidney essence.

RIGHT **Menopausal problems can be related to weakness in Kidney energies and *Jing*.**

Additional treatments for menopausal syndrome might involve acupuncture at points like RM4 (*Guanyuan*), RM3 (*Zhongji*), or SP6 (*Sanyinjiao*). Typically, treatment would be given on a daily basis for three weeks.

RIGHT **Traditionally, silver acupuncture needles were used to stimulate yin, and gold ones for yang.**

RIGHT **Moxa** sticks are sliced and used in moxabustion to warm cold conditions.

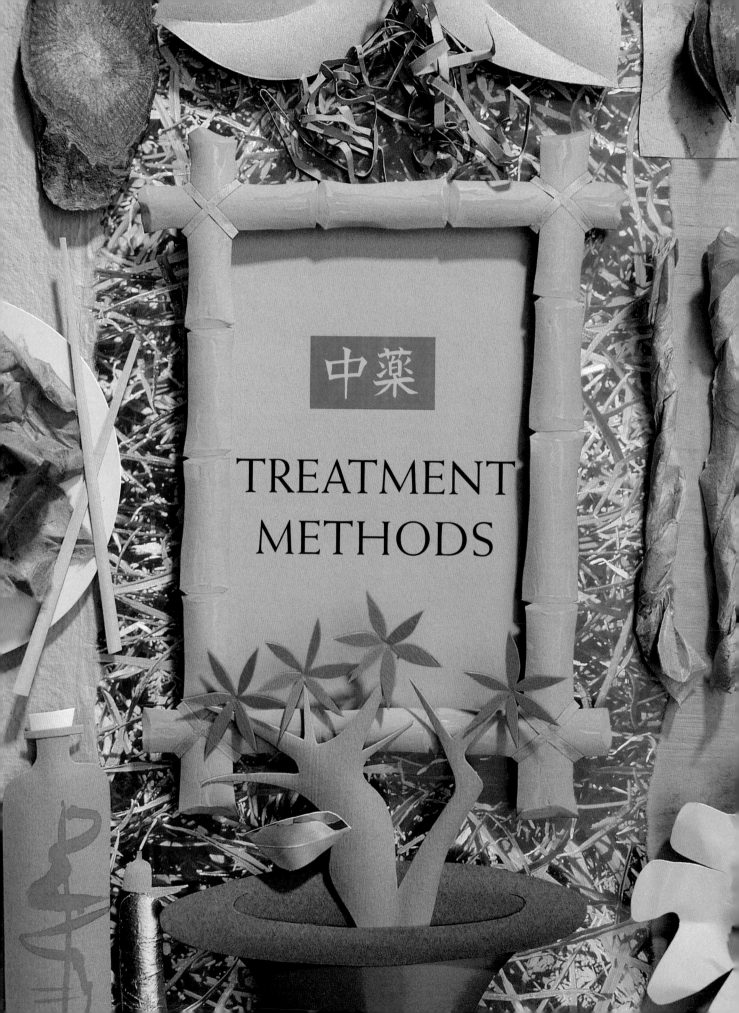

中藥

TREATMENT
METHODS

CHINESE HERBAL MEDICINE

I n the West, herbs tend to be thought of as useful plants that can be used in cooking and medicine, or may be valued as aromatics for perfumery. In traditional Chinese medicine, the concept of "herb" is very different and is better translated as "drug."

MORE THAN JUST PLANTS

As any Western herbal written before the 17th century shows, early Western physicians agreed with the Chinese that healing "herbs" included far more than the modern concept of hedgerow plants and aromatic garden flowers. The 16th-century *Grete Herbal* includes "mummy" from decomposing corpses as a suitable remedy, while as late as 1640 John Parkinson was still enthusing about the therapeutic properties of the unicorn's horn, and, to the 18th-century doctor, arsenic and antimony were valuable medicines.

Traditional Chinese medicine is no different, and the "herbs" listed in a typical *materia medica* will include animal parts, insects, and crushed ores. The "herbs" are listed not by the botanical name of the growing plant, as is usual in the West, but by the name of the prepared or dried "drug." Different parts of the same plant go under different names, and the labels change again if the dried plant is stir-fried or treated with ginger before use. Even more confusing for Westerners, the same "drug" can be derived from a number of different botanical species, depending on where in the vast spaces of China it is collected.

The properties of these different plant parts and preparations also vary.

Rou Gui, for example, is cinnamon bark (from *Cinnamomum cassia*), largely used to tonify Kidney yang and dispel cold, while *Gui Zhi* is the twigs from the same tree used as a diaphoretic to warm the channels and encourage blood circulation. To add to the confusion, *Gui Pi* is the bark of a different type of cinnamon tree (usually *C. japonicum*), used to warm the Spleen and Stomach, and also improve circulation.

CHINESE PRESCRIPTIONS

It is rare for a Chinese prescription to comprise only one or two herbs; usually four or more are combined in a traditional formula which often dates back to the earliest practitioners and classics like **Jingui Yaolue (The Prescriptions of the Golden Chamber)** by Zhang Zhongjing (c.150–219 CE). Chinese medical students learn thousands of these formulae by heart in their training, each one a specific remedy for an exactly defined disease syndrome.

Within the prescription, each herb also has a precise role:
• Emperor – the principal therapeutic herbs
• Minister – herbs that support and strengthen the key plants
• Messenger – based on the directional properties of the plants to

"target" the prescription to particular meridians or parts of the body
• Helper or harmonizer – auxiliary and/or correcting herbs which can counter any toxic effects of the major ingredients or deal with secondary symptoms in the condition.

The prescriptions may be used as a standard remedy or modified to suit the individual. In the West, some of the most popular combinations are prepacked in tablets or as powdered mixtures, and these are often supplied by acupuncturists as a convenient remedy. Herbalists generally prefer to blend the raw herbs, adjusting the mixture to suit the patient.

HERB PART NAMES

Translating Chinese terms into English is never easy, as subtle changes in pronunciation of apparently the same word alter the meaning dramatically; these herb part names are, however, reasonably consistent:

Hua	flower
Pi	bark
Teng	stem
Ye	leaf
Zhi	twig or branch
Zi	fruit

CLASSIC CHARACTERISTICS OF HERBS

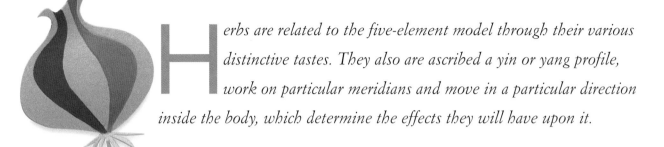

Herbs are related to the five-element model through their various distinctive tastes. They also are ascribed a yin or yang profile, work on particular meridians and move in a particular direction inside the body, which determine the effects they will have upon it.

DIFFERENT DEFINITIONS

As in traditional Western herbal medicine, Chinese theory assesses healing plants in terms of the effects they have on the body – cooling or heating, drying or moistening. These properties are largely determined by the taste of the plant and its characteristic yin–yang profile.

Instead of describing plants in such modern medical terms as antibacterial or anti-inflammatory, a typical Chinese herbal will instead provide details of:
• the plant's "property" – whether the plant is hot/warm, neutral, or cool/cold
• its "taste" – matching the classic five tastes of pungent, sweet, sour, bitter, and salty and adding two further options – astringent or bland/neutral
• which of the main channels or meridians it affects or "enters", and sometimes also
• its "direction" once inside the body – whether lifting, lowering, floating, or sinking.

RIGHT **Chinese herbs are used to counterbalance symptoms of disease and restore the body's harmony.**

PROPERTIES

As with "Galenical medicine," which was practiced in Europe until well into the 17th century, Chinese herbs are used to counterbalance the symptoms of the disease. A fever or other illness that involves heat, for example, would be treated with a cold herb, while something that involves cold – such as osteoarthritis or watery catarrh – would be treated by a heating herb.

Huang Qin (*Scutellaria baicalensis*), for example, is classified as a cold herb and is used to treat a range of disorders involving heat or characterized by fever, thirst, rapid pulse rate, and a red tongue with a yellow coating.

In contrast, *Shan Yao* (*Dioscorea opposita*) is a neutral remedy, not specifically hot or cold, so it can be suitable for a wider range of symptoms.

PROPERTIES AND SYNDROMES

Property	Action	Syndrome
Cold/cool	To clear Heat	Heat syndromes
	To purge Fire	Yang syndromes
	To remove toxins	Heat toxin syndromes
Warm/hot	To warm the interior	Cold syndromes
	To dispel Cold evils	Yin syndromes
	To strengthen yang	Yang deficient syndrome
Neutral	Milder actions, so may both clear heat and warm the interior, etc.	All syndromes

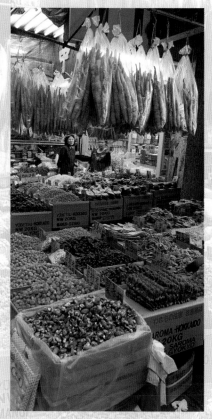

ABOVE **Traditional herb suppliers in China offer an enormous variety of medicinal plants.**

TASTES

Each of the five tastes has its own particular effect on the body and is related to the five-element model. Therefore, in some cases, those tastes should be avoided if the associated organ is affected.

Sweet tastes, for example, can be especially damaging in cases of stagnation and Damp affecting the Spleen and Stomach, while salty tastes will increase edema and water retention because of their effect on the Kidneys.

TASTES AND SYNDROMES

Taste	Action	Syndrome/symptoms
Pungent	Dispersing	Superficial syndrome Wind syndrome
	Mobilizing	Stagnant *Qi* syndrome Stagnant Blood syndrome
Sour and astringent	Contracting	Sweating associated with deficiency Hemorrhage due to deficiency Chronic diarrhea Enuresis
Sweet	Tonifying	Yin, yang, or *Qi* deficient syndrome
	Alleviating Clearing toxins Harmonizing the action of drugs	Spasmodic pain
Salty	Softening and eliminating	Combating swellings (e.g., in the lymphatic system) and other masses
	Lubricating the Large Intestine	Constipation
Bitter	Reversing the upward motion of *Qi*	Coughs, vomiting Constipation due to stagnation Problems with urination
	Drying damp evils Activating *Qi* and Blood motion	Water–Damp syndromes Coughs due to stagnant Lung *Qi* Stagnant Blood syndromes
Bland	Diuresis	Water–Damp syndromes

MERIDIAN

Each herb is believed to affect particular channels most strongly, so the remedy of choice will be one which has an affinity with the appropriate channel for the affected organs.

Jie Geng (*Platycodon grandiflorum*), for example, is a very effective cough remedy, which has a particular affinity with the Lung channel (*see* page 29) (*Hand Tai Yin*). *Ju Hua* (*Dendranthema* x *grandiflorum*) has a similar affinity with the Lung channel. It is used to treat the coughs and congestion which accompany superficial Wind–Heat syndrome (a feverish common cold), but it also has a connection to the Liver channel (*Foot Jue Yin*) and is helpful for various disorders associated with Liver Heat, such as conjunctivitis.

DIRECTION

As with properties, the Chinese physician will choose herbs which have a counter direction to the characteristics of the disease syndrome: illnesses which have a tendency to rise through the body would, therefore, be treated with herbs which are lowering or sinking. Constipation, for example, where the upward trend is countering the normal stool movement, would be treated by a sinking herb – such as *Da Huang* (*Rheum palmatum*).

In a variant on the Western Doctrine of Signatures tradition, herbal tendencies are typified by the appearance and part of the plant used – flowers, leaves and fur are likely to be lifting or floating, while seeds, fruits, and minerals fall to the ground, and therefore are considered to be lowering or sinking.

Roots and rhizomes may be included in either category – as you might well appreciate by comparing rhizomes and tubers that tend to grow horizontally with tap roots that tend to go down.

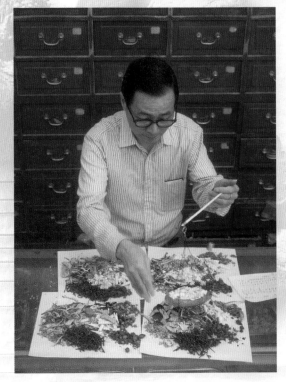

RIGHT **Herbs are traditionally dispensed in bags containing enough for a single dose.**

DIRECTION AND ACTION		
Tendency	**Action**	**Syndrome**
Lifting/ floating	Upward and outward as in: • lifting yang • inducing sweating • expelling cold evils	Headaches; superficial syndromes; prolapse
Lowering/ sinking	Down and inward as in: • suppressing *yang* • reversing the upward flow of *Qi* • as an astringent • clearing heat evils • eliminating dampness • purging	Constipation; difficulties with urination; Interior Heat syndrome; Interior Cold syndrome; cough; vomiting

TAKING CHINESE HERBS

raditionally, most Chinese medicines are taken in soups or decoctions – brewed in a large crock pot kept specially for the purpose and drunk from steaming soup bowls each morning.

BREWING THE *TANG*

Although many Westernized products are now appearing in Chinese herbal shops, most still sell the same assortment of crude dried roots, barks, and flowers familiar for generations. Patients take their prescriptions to the herbal dispensary where the list of dried herbs is assembled in separate paper bags, enough in each for a single dose. This is traditionally boiled in three cups of water in an earthenware or ceramic pot for 25–30 minutes until the liquid has reduced by half. The mixture is then strained and taken in a single dose on an empty stomach in the morning. The same herbs might be used for the following day's brew, depending on the exact mix. If it contains soluble ingredients, such as certain mineral salts, then a fresh prescription will be needed each day.

The soup (*Tang*) is generally dark brown and strongly flavored. Chinese doses are larger than Western doses – often up to 3oz (90g) – and the resulting mix is usually too strongly flavored for Western palates.

PILLS AND POWDERS

Simpler to take are the powders and pills which are ready-made and simply need to be measured each day. The dose of a powdered mixture is generally stirred into half a cup of warm water, while pills are traditionally made from ground herbs blended with honey and rolled into pellets.

Modern demands for more convenient potions are starting to change some of the traditional brews. Prescriptions that were traditionally made into soups, such as *Si Jun Zi Tang*, are now available in ready-mixed powdered concentrations or Western-style tinctures and can be taken in a simple teaspoon dose stirred into water. Although there is little difference in the powdered and crude herbs, some traditional Chinese practitioners believe that changing the style of the formulation could affect its therapeutics. The Western fondness for tinctures as a convenient extract, for example, produces a brew containing alcohol – itself used as a warming therapeutic ingredient in some Chinese formulae – so these mixtures could be more heating than the original soups, pills or powders.

Wines (*see* pages 112–113) are also traditionally used in tonic brews, with a large vat filled with a tonic herb such as *Dang Gui* (*Angelica polyphorma* var. *sinensis*), *He Shou Wu* (*Polygonum multiflorum*), or *Ren Shen* (*Panax ginseng*), and then covered with wine. The mixture is left for a few weeks and then doses of it taken on a daily basis. According to one legend, the sage Li Ch'ing Yuen, reputedly born in 1678 in Southwest China, died in 1930 at the age of 252 years, after surviving 14 wives, with the help of a small glass of mixed *He Shou Wu* and *Ren Shen* tonic wine taken each evening before bed.

PREPARATIONS

Chinese herbs are taken in one of the following forms:

Jiu	wine
San	powder
Tang	decoction/soup
Wan	pill

A HOMOEOPATHIC REMEDY

PREPARED HERBS

Western herbal medicine generally uses herbs in either their crude/fresh or dried states, but in China there are far more options, as herbs can be stir-fried, cooked with wine or vinegar, and steamed or processed with salt or ginger. These different treatments are believed to subtly alter the properties of the plants.

Magnolia bark (*Hou Po*), for example, is mixed with ginger juice to make it warmer and more pungent so that its "lifting/floating" tendency may help to mobilize *Qi*. Once fried with wine, *Huang Qin* (*Scutellaria baicalensis*) – generally used to clear heat and dampness from the Lung – becomes *Jiu Zhi Huang Qin*, with the added pungency of the wine increasing its uplifting action and making it a more effective expectorant.

In contrast, the sourness of vinegar adds an astringent taste, and sourness also focuses action on the Liver channel, giving the herb more of a lowering/sinking action. Adding a pinch of salt to particular decoctions also changes the dominant taste, focusing attention downward and on the Kidneys.

Processing can also help to reduce toxicity. Aconite (*Aconitum carmichaeli*) is an extremely poisonous plant that is legally restricted to external use in Western herbal medicine. By cooking it with salt, sugar, and sulfur, Chinese herbalists convert it into a safe remedy – *Fu Zi* – which is used in cases of shock and severe cold syndromes.

EASE POWDER

XIAO YAO SAN

Chai Hu (Bupleurum chinense) 30g
Dang Gui (Angelica polyphorma var. sinensis) 30g
Bai Zhu (Atractylodes macrocephala) 30g
Bai Shao (Paeonia lactiflora) 30g
Fu Ling (Wolfiporia cocos) 30g
Gan Cao (Glycyrrhiza uralensis) 15g

Xiao Yao San is one of the most popular combinations for coordinating Liver and Spleen function and relieving stagnant Liver energy – seen in Chinese medicine as a key cause of what in the West is termed "premenstrual syndrome" (PMS). About 6–9g of the powdered ingredients are traditionally taken at each dose, with the addition of a tiny amount (1–3g) of *Bo He* (*Mentha arvensis*) and *Sheng Jiang* (*Zingiber officinale*) decoction, as this is believed to be a more effective way of taking the herbs. Modern pre-prepared Ease Powder preparations combine all the ingredients in a single, convenient brew.

THE FOUR NOBLE INGREDIENTS DECOCTION

SI JUN ZI TANG

Ren Shen (Panax ginseng) 12g
Bai Zhu (Atractylodes macrocephala) 9g
Fu Ling (Wolfiporia cocos) 9g
Gan Cao (Glycyrrhiza uralensis) 4.5g

This is one of the great classic formulations of Chinese medicine – used as a tonic mix to replenish *Qi*, invigorate the Middle *Jiao* and tonify Spleen and Stomach. It is used whenever there is obvious Spleen/Stomach weakness, such as in chronic gastroenteritis and duodenal ulceration. *Gan Cao* acts as the harmonizing herb, while *Ren Shen* and *Bai Zhu* are the key tonic herbs, supported by *Fu Ling*; all three enter the Spleen channel. Today, it is available ready-made in the West as a tincture mixture or concentrated powdered extract – quite different from the traditional concept of a soup.

BELOW **Most Chinese medicines are taken in the form of *Tang* (soup or decoction).**

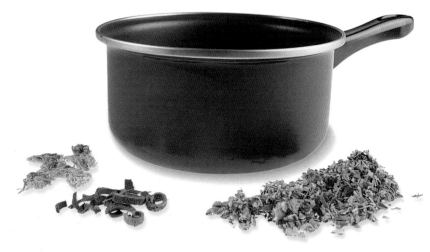

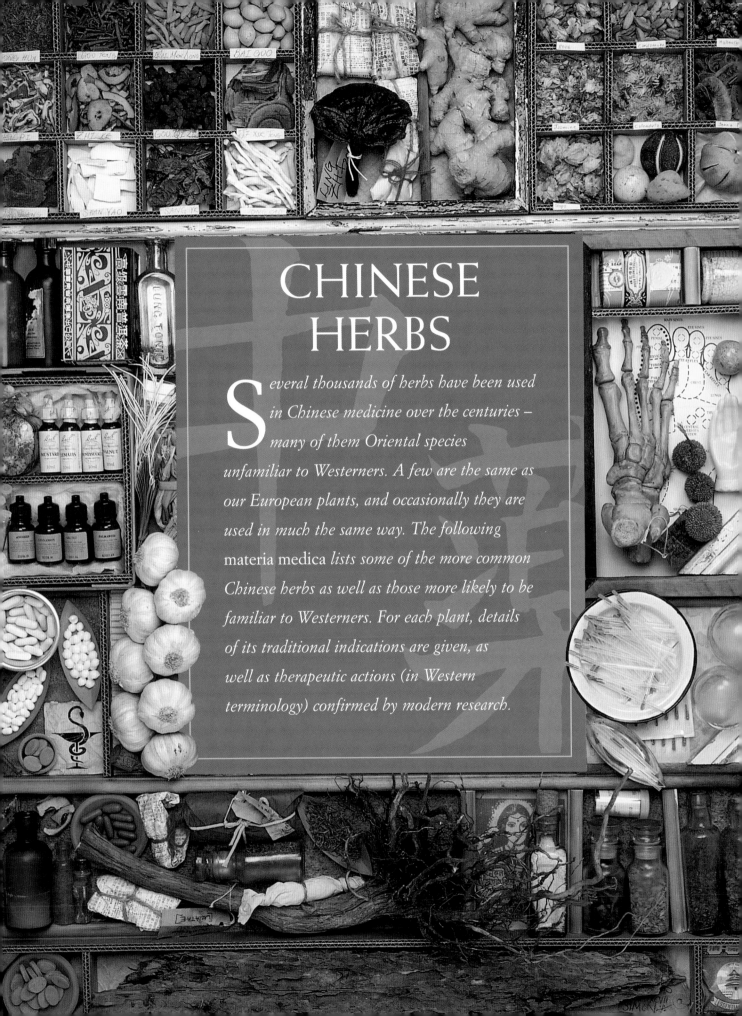

CHINESE HERBS

Several thousands of herbs have been used in Chinese medicine over the centuries – many of them Oriental species unfamiliar to Westerners. A few are the same as our European plants, and occasionally they are used in much the same way. The following materia medica *lists some of the more common Chinese herbs as well as those more likely to be familiar to Westerners. For each plant, details of its traditional indications are given, as well as therapeutic actions (in Western terminology) confirmed by modern research.*

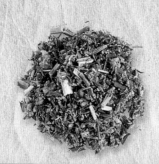

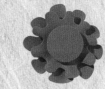

AI YE

PARTS USED
Leaves
TASTE
Pungent, bitter
CHARACTER
Warm
MERIDIANS
*Lung, Liver, Spleen,
Kidney*

BOTANICAL NAME
Artemisia vulgaris
COMMON NAME
Mugwort

Mugwort is a familiar wayside plant in Europe, and was once associated with magic and witchcraft. In China, it is the *moxa* used for moxabustion treatments (*see* pages 92–93) and is also an important gynecological remedy. Studies suggest that, like its relative *Artemisia annua* (*Qing Hao*), it combats malaria.

ACTIONS
antibacterial, antifungal, expectorant, uterine stimulant

INDICATIONS
☻ to warm the meridians
☻ to stop bleeding
☻ to dispel Cold and pain
☻ to resolve Phlegm in coughs/asthma

USES
Ai Ye is largely used for menstrual problems, including menorrhagia and painful menstruation. It is said to "calm the fetus" and has been used for threatened miscarriage and infertility. It is combined with *Gan Jiang* or *Rou Gui* for abdominal pain linked with Cold.

BAI SHAO

PARTS USED
Root
TASTE
Sour, bitter
CHARACTER
Slightly cold
MERIDIANS
Liver, Spleen

BOTANICAL NAME
Paeonia lactiflora
COMMON NAME
White peony

Use of white peony root dates back to about 500 CE when it was listed in Tao Hong-jing's *Ben Cao Jing Ji Zhu*. It is mainly used as a nourishing Blood tonic and for Liver disharmonies, so is a popular gynecological herb. *Bai Shao* is roasted to reduce its cold nature.

ACTIONS
antibacterial, anti-inflammatory, antispasmodic, diuretic, sedative, hypotensive, analgesic

INDICATIONS
☻ to balance Liver functions and energy
☻ to nourish Blood and consolidate yin
☻ to soothe Liver Qi and relieve pain

USES
It is used for a wide range of problems associated with Blood deficiency and Liver Qi problems, including ascending Liver yang (typified by headaches and dizziness) and disharmonies between Spleen and Liver, when it is often used with *Gan Cao*. It is combined with *Dang Gui* and *Shu Di Huang* for menstrual problems.

BAI ZHU

PARTS USED
Rhizome
TASTE
Sweet, bitter
CHARACTER
Warm
MERIDIANS
Spleen, Stomach

BOTANICAL NAME
*Atractylodes
macrocephala*
COMMON NAME
White atractylodes

Bai Zhu is one of the main *Qi* tonics used especially for Spleen or Stomach Qi deficiency syndromes. The herb has been used in China since the Tang Dynasty (c.650 CE). It is included in the famous *Si Jun Zi Tang* ("Four Noble Ingredients Decoction") – an important energy-giving brew (*see* pages 56–57).

ACTIONS
antibacterial, anticoagulant, digestive stimulant, diuretic, hypoglycemic

INDICATIONS
☻ to tonify the Spleen and *Qi*
☻ to clear Dampness
☻ to control excess sweating and strengthen resistance

USES
Bai Zhu is mainly used for problems associated with Spleen or Stomach deficiency with such typical symptoms as diarrhea, tiredness, abdominal bloating, poor appetite, and nausea. It is also said to "dry Dampness" and is used for edema and fluid retention.

CONTRAINDICATIONS
Avoid in epileptics. Use in pregnancy only under professional guidance.

CONTRAINDICATIONS
Avoid in cases of diarrhea and abdominal coldness.

CONTRAINDICATIONS
Avoid in yin deficiency characterized by extreme thirst.

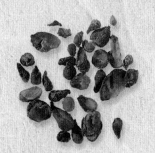
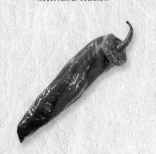
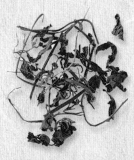

BAN XIA

PARTS USED
Tuber
TASTE
Pungent
CHARACTER
Warm
MERIDIANS
Lung, Spleen, Stomach

BOTANICAL NAME
Pinellia ternata
COMMON NAME
Pinellia

Ban Xia literally means "half summer" because the herb is traditionally collected at midsummer. It was one of the herbs listed in the *Shen Nong Ben Cao Jing.* It is a toxic plant and is usually soaked in tea or vinegar before use.

ACTIONS
antiemetic, antitussive, expectorant, lowers blood cholesterol levels; one study suggests it may relieve toothache

INDICATIONS
◉ to clear Phlegm and Dampness
◉ to disperse lumps and swellings
◉ to reverse the flow of *Qi*

USES
Ban Xia is one of the herbs which "transforms cold Phlegm" – it clears Dampness, especially Damp Spleen, will cause rebellious *Qi* to descend and harmonizes the Stomach to stop vomiting. Rising *Qi* is seen in Chinese medicine as a cause of productive coughing. *Fa Ban Xia* is combined with alum, licorice, and calcium carbonate as a Phlegm remedy.

BI BA

PARTS USED
Fruit spikes
TASTE
Pungent
CHARACTER
Hot
MERIDIANS
Spleen, Stomach

BOTANICAL NAME
Piper longum
COMMON NAME
Indian long pepper, pippali

Pippali is important in Ayurvedic medicine as a remedy for colds, bronchitis, arthritis, lumbago, indigestion, and wind. In China, it is mainly used as a very warming remedy for stomach chills and vomiting. It was first listed in China in the 10th century in the *Kai Bao Ben Cao* and was possibly introduced by Buddhist monks then arriving from India.

ACTIONS
antibacterial

INDICATIONS
◉ to warm the abdomen and dispel Cold
◉ to reverse the flow of *Qi*
◉ to relieve pain

USES
Bi Ba is used for Cold Stomach syndromes which are characterized by nausea, abdominal pain, and chills. A powder of the herb is used as a topical remedy for toothache. It is used with herbs like *Dang Shen, Rou Gui,* and *Gan Jiang* for diarrhea associated with Cold.

BO HE

PARTS USED
Aerial parts
TASTE
Pungent
CHARACTER
Cool
MERIDIANS
Liver, Lung

BOTANICAL NAME
Mentha arvensis
COMMON NAME
Field mint

Field mint is traditionally used in the West in tea, and to prevent milk from curdling. The oil is sometimes added as an adulterant to peppermint oil. The Chinese mainly use *Bo He* as a remedy for superficial "Wind–Heat" problems – such as feverish colds and skin eruptions.

ACTIONS
antibacterial, anti-inflammatory, antispasmodic, analgesic, diaphoretic

INDICATIONS
◉ to disperse Wind and Heat evils
◉ to clear the head and give good spirit
◉ to encourage the eruption of skin rashes, as in measles
◉ to disperse stagnant Liver *Qi* and relieve depression

USES
Bo He is used to relieve feverish chills with slight sweating, body pains, and headache, as in the early stages of flu; in the early stages of infections associated with irritant rashes; and for pain in the chest linked to Liver stagnation.

CONTRAINDICATIONS
Avoid in pregnancy and Blood disorders.

CONTRAINDICATIONS
Not to be used if there are Fire symptoms or Heat caused by yin deficiency.

CONTRAINDICATIONS
Avoid in yin deficiency and excess Liver *Qi.*

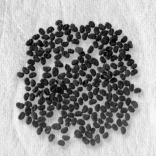

BU GU ZHI

PARTS USED
Fruit and seeds
TASTE
Pungent, bitter
CHARACTER
Very warm
MERIDIANS
Kidney, Spleen

BOTANICAL NAME
Psoralea corylifolia
COMMON NAME
Malay tea, scurf pea, scuffy pea

Bu Gu Zhi is one of the main tonic herbs for yang. It is particularly effective for Kidney energies. Traditionally, it is used for "cock crow diarrhea" – loose stools in the early morning which are characteristic of Spleen and Kidney yang deficiency.

ACTIONS
antibacterial, antitumor, astringent, uterine stimulant, vasodilator for the coronary arteries, increases skin photosensitivity

INDICATIONS
☙ to reinforce Kidney yang
☙ to warm Spleen yang

USES
Bu Gu Zhi is used for Kidney yang deficiency, which is likely to be typified by impotence, lower back pain, or urinary incontinence. For cock crow diarrhea, it is often combined with *Rou Dou Kou, Wu Wei Zhi,* and *Wu Zhu Yu.* For back pain associated with Kidney yang deficiency, it can be used with *Hu Tao Ren.*

> **CONTRAINDICATIONS**
> Not to be used if there is deficient yin or excess Fire.

CANG ER ZI

PARTS USED
Fruit
TASTE
Pungent, bitter
CHARACTER
Warm, toxic
MERIDIANS
Lung

BOTANICAL NAME
Xanthium strumarium
COMMON NAME
Cocklebur

Cang Er Zi literally means "deep green ear seeds" and it is one of the herbs used to clear Wind–Damp. Typically Wind–Damp leads to nasal congestion, and studies in China have shown that the herb is a very effective anticatarrhal.

ACTIONS
antibacterial, antifungal, antirheumatic, antispasmodic, analgesic. It contains a chemical called xanthostrumarin which may be toxic in high doses and lead to convulsions.

INDICATIONS
☙ to open the nasal passages
☙ to dispel Wind–Damp – including *Bi* syndrome (arthritis) and skin irritations
☙ to relieve pain due to exterior Wind

USES
Cang Er Zi is ideal for colds and chills characterized by headaches, aching limbs, and nasal congestion. It is often combined with *Xin Yi, Bo He,* and *Jin Yin Hua* for sinus problems, or with *Jin Ying Zi* and *Wu Wei Zi* for allergic rhinitis.

> **CONTRAINDICATIONS**
> Not to be used for headache or arthritic pains associated with anemia or Blood deficiency.

CANG ZHU

PARTS USED
Rhizome
TASTE
Pungent, bitter
CHARACTER
Warm
MERIDIANS
Spleen, Stomach

BOTANICAL NAME
Atractylodes chinensis
COMMON NAME
Gray atractylodes

Cang Zhu is one of the main herbs for clearing Dampness – both for internal Damp problems associated with the Spleen, and for external Damp. The famous 16th-century herbalist Li Shi Zhen recommended fumigation with *Cang Zhu* during epidemics as an important preventive.

ACTIONS
carminative, diaphoretic, increases excretion of sodium and potassium salts, although it is not diuretic.

INDICATIONS
☙ dries Dampness and tonifies the Spleen
☙ expels external Wind, Damp and Cold
☙ clears Dampness in the *San Jiao*

USES
Cang Zhu is used for a range of digestive problems associated with Damp in the Spleen or Middle/Lower *Jiao,* including nausea, vomiting, indigestion, and diarrhea. It is often combined with *Hou Po* or *Xiang Fu.* The herb is also used for arthritic problems and is a traditional remedy for night blindness.

> **CONTRAINDICATIONS**
> Not to be used in *Qi* or yin deficiency associated with Interior Heat.

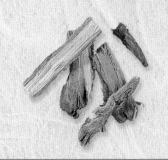
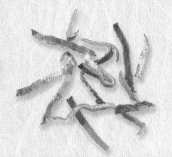
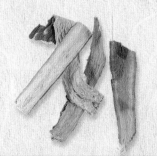

CHAI HU

PARTS USED
Root
TASTE
Bitter, pungent
CHARACTER
Slightly cold
MERIDIANS
Liver, Gall bladder, San Jiao, Pericardium

BOTANICAL NAME
Bupleurum chinense
COMMON NAME
Thorowax

Although *Chai Hu* is generally regarded as a remedy for fevers and chills, it is also a potent Liver herb and Western herbalists sometimes liken it to vervain (*Verbena officinalis*). Related species are popular in the West for flower arrangements and as a garden ornamental.

ACTIONS
antibacterial, antiviral, antimalarial, analgesic, anti-inflammatory, cholagogue, mild hypotensive, sedative

INDICATIONS
☺ to disperse Wind and Heat evils
☺ to disperse stagnant Liver *Qi* and relieve depression
☺ to raise yang *Qi* and combat prolapse

USES
Chai Hu is used for feverish colds, malaria, and similar conditions associated with feverishness, dizziness, and chest pains. It is popular for clearing stagnant Liver *Qi*, which can cause menstrual problems and depression, as well as for Damp affecting the Liver meridian.

CHEN PI

PARTS USED
Peel
TASTE
Pungent, bitter
CHARACTER
Warm
MERIDIANS
Lung, Spleen, Stomach

BOTANICAL NAME
Citrus reticulata
COMMON NAME
Tangerine, mandarin orange

Chen Pi is included in Shen Nong's original herbal; it is the orange-colored peel of ripe tangerines. Other tangerine remedies are *Qing Pi*, the peel from unripe green fruits, and *Ju He* (the seed). *Qing Pi* focuses on the Liver and Gall Bladder, while *Ju He* is used for the Liver and Kidneys.

ACTIONS
antiasthmatic, anti-inflammatory, carminative, digestive stimulant, expectorant, circulatory stimulant; the plant is also effective for acute mastitis

INDICATIONS
☺ to strengthen and move stagnant Spleen and Stomach *Qi*
☺ to dry Dampness and resolve Phlegm
☺ to reverse the upward flow of *Qi*
☺ to help prevent stagnation, especially when using tonifying herbs

USES
It eases abdominal discomfort and poor appetite and is an effective expectorant for coughs with thick copious sputum. It reverses rising *Qi* associated with vomiting.

CHI SHAO

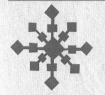

PARTS USED
Root
TASTE
Sour, bitter
CHARACTER
Slightly cold
MERIDIANS
Liver, Spleen

BOTANICAL NAME
Paeonia lactiflora
COMMON NAME
Red peony

Red peony has been used in China since at least 500 CE. It is one of the main Blood stimulants, helping the circulation and clearing stagnation. As a cooling remedy, it is a specific for Hot Blood syndromes.

ACTIONS
antibacterial, anti-inflammatory, anticoagulant, immune stimulant, lowers Blood cholesterol, peripheral vasodilator, hypoglycemic, sedative, stimulates tissue repair, improves microcirculation

INDICATIONS
☺ to invigorate Blood and dispel Blood stagnation
☺ to clear Heat and cool the Blood
☺ to clear Liver Fire

USES
Chi Shao is used for menstrual pains, and for scanty periods and abdominal pain due to Blood stagnation. It cools Blood so it is sometimes included in prescriptions for skin problems – it was used in a trial of Chinese remedies for children with severe eczema at a London Hospital.

CONTRAINDICATIONS
Avoid in cases of Liver Fire or yin deficiency.

CONTRAINDICATIONS
Avoid if there is hemoptysis or no sign of Damp/Phlegm stagnation.

CONTRAINDICATIONS
Avoid if there is no evidence of Blood stagnation.

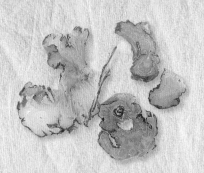

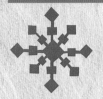

CHUAN XIONG

PARTS USED
Rhizome
TASTE
Pungent
CHARACTER
Warm
MERIDIANS
*Liver, Pericardium,
Gall Bladder*

BOTANICAL NAME
Ligusticum wallichii
COMMON NAME
*Sichuan or Szechuan
lovage*

Chuan Xiong is related to both
European lovage, largely used as a
culinary herb, and osha
(*L. porteri*), a popular North
American herb. It has been used in
China since the 14th century for
menstrual and Heart problems.

ACTIONS
antibacterial, hypotensive, sedative, uterine
stimulant

INDICATIONS
☺ to invigorate the circulation of Blood
and *Qi*
☺ to relieve pain, headache, and skin
eruptions caused by Wind
☺ moves the *Qi* upward

USES
It is combined with *Dang Gui*, *Bai Shao*,
and *Shu Di Huang* for menstrual
irregularities and anemia (in *Si Wu Tang* or
"four ingredients decoction"). *Chuan
Xiong* is also used with a variety of other
herbs to treat headaches due to Wind,
Heat, Cold, or Deficient Blood. It is also
used for coronary heart disease.

CONG BAI

PARTS USED
Bulb
TASTE
Pungent
CHARACTER
Warm
MERIDIAN
Lung, Stomach

BOTANICAL NAME
Allium fistulosum
COMMON NAME
*Scallion/spring
onion*

Cong Bai – familiar as a salad
vegetable in the West – shares
many properties with its relatives:
garlic, ramsons (wild garlic), and
onion, which are all used in Western
herbal medicine.

ACTIONS
antibacterial, antifungal, diaphoretic,
diuretic, expectorant

INDICATIONS
☺ to dispel Wind and Cold evils
☺ to invigorate yang *Qi*

USES:
Cong Bai is used in the early stages of
common colds when there is a chill, cough,
and nasal catarrh. It is also helpful for
abdominal chills and bloating, or where
there are problems from extreme cold –
such as in frostbite.

DA HUANG

PARTS USED
Root and rhizome
TASTE
Bitter
CHARACTER
Cold
MERIDIANS
*Liver, Spleen,
Stomach, Large
Intestine*

BOTANICAL NAME
Rheum palmatum
COMMON NAME
*Turkey rhubarb,
Chinese rhubarb*

Da Huang – which means "big
yellow" in Chinese (from the
color of its root) – is used mainly as a
purgative, as it is in traditional
Western herbal treatments.

ACTIONS
purgative, antibacterial, antifungal,
antiparasitic, hypotensive, lowers blood
cholesterol levels, cholagogue, diuretic

INDICATIONS
☺ to drain Heat including Damp–Heat and
excess Heat in the Blood
☺ to invigorate Blood circulation and clear
Blood stagnation
☺ to detoxify Fire poison

USES
Da Huang is used for fevers associated
with constipation and abdominal fullness,
and for Heat in the Blood where
symptoms may include nosebleeds or
bleeding piles. It is used in jaundice and
acute infections as a detoxificant, and
externally for boils and suppurating skin
diseases. It clears stagnant Blood, and may
be given for irregular menstruation.

CONTRAINDICATIONS
Avoid in cases of headache caused by
yin deficiency/overexuberant Liver
yang, and pregnancy or menorrhagia.

CONTRAINDICATIONS
Avoid where there is
spontaneous sweating.

CONTRAINDICATIONS
Avoid if there are no Heat
or Fire symptoms.

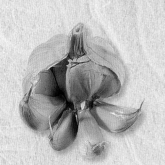
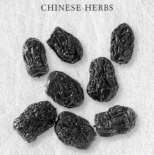
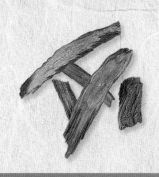

DA SUAN

PARTS USED
Bulb
TASTE
Pungent
CHARACTER
Warm
MERIDIANS
Spleen, Stomach, Lung, Large Intestine

BOTANICAL NAME
Allium sativum
COMMON NAME
Garlic

While garlic is used in the West as both an antimicrobial and an anticholesterol remedy for the Heart and circulatory system, the Chinese view it in far narrower terms as an antiparasitic remedy. It is sometimes combined with *Da Huang* as a poultice for acute abscesses.

ACTIONS
antiparasitic, antibiotic, expectorant, diaphoretic, hypotensive, antithrombotic, reduces cholesterol levels, hypoglycemic

INDICATIONS
- kills parasites
- detoxifies poisons

USES
Garlic is used in China for treating hookworm, pinworms, and other sorts of intestinal parasites. It is also used externally for ringworm and may be taken internally for dysentery. The garlic cloves are generally eaten raw or may be made into a garlic congee (*see* page 110) – a traditional remedy for severe chest problems such as tuberculosis.

DA ZAO

PARTS USED
Fruit
TASTE
Sweet
CHARACTER
Warm
MERIDIANS
Spleen, Stomach

BOTANICAL NAME
Ziziphus jujuba
COMMON NAME
Chinese dates, jujube

Da Zao literally means "big date" and the fruits are one of the important "harmonizers" of Chinese medicine, often added – like licorice (*Gan Cao*) – to prescriptions to help modify and blend any conflicts in the action of the different ingredients.

ACTIONS
nutrient, protects against liver damage

INDICATIONS
- to tonify Spleen and Stomach *Qi*
- to strengthen nourishing *Qi* (ying *Qi*) and Blood
- to calm the spirit (*Shen*)
- to moderate the action of other herbs

USES
The usual method of taking *Da Zao* is to add three to ten dates to the *Tang*. The dates are often used for general debility and lack of appetite associated with Spleen *Qi* deficiency. It is used in anemia to help nourish Blood and is also regarded as calming *Shen* so may be given for palpitations and irritability associated with deficient Heart energy.

DAN SHEN

PARTS USED
Root and rhizome
TASTE
Bitter
CHARACTER
Slightly cold
MERIDIANS
Heart, Liver, Pericardium

BOTANICAL NAME
Salvia miltiorrhiza
COMMON NAME
Chinese sage, red sage

Chinese sage is an important Heart and Blood remedy, which has been shown in clinical trials to help both Heart disease and problems with cerebral circulation. It is used with *Tan Xiang* and *Sha Ren* in the prescription *Dan Shen Yin*, for angina pectoris.

ACTIONS
anticoagulant, antibacterial, immune stimulant, circulatory stimulant, peripheral vasodilator, promotes tissue repair, sedative, lowers blood cholesterol

INDICATIONS
- to invigorate the Blood circulation and clear Blood stagnation
- to clear Heat
- to calm the spirit and soothe irritability

USES
As it affects the Liver meridian, *Dan Shen* is – not surprisingly – used for period pains and irregular or scanty menstruation. It is an important herb for Heart disease as well as for insomnia and palpitations, related to deficient Heart Blood.

CONTRAINDICATIONS
Avoid in deficient yin patterns with Heat signs.

CONTRAINDICATIONS
Avoid in cases of excessive Dampness, food stagnation, or Phlegm.

CONTRAINDICATIONS
Avoid if there is no Blood stagnation.

DANG GUI

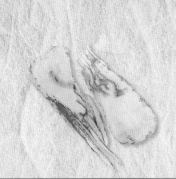

PARTS USED
Root
TASTE
Sweet, pungent
CHARACTER
Warm
BOTANICAL NAME
Angelica polyphorma var. *sinensis*
COMMON NAME
Chinese angelica
MERIDIANS
Liver, Heart, Spleen

Dang Gui is one of the most popular Chinese tonic herbs available in the West. Different parts of the root have different qualities – the bottom tip is said to move Blood most strongly, while the uppermost part is a stronger tonic.

ACTIONS
antibacterial, analgesic, anti-inflammatory, circulatory stimulant, reduces blood cholesterol levels, liver tonic, sedative, uterine stimulant, rich in B vitamins

INDICATIONS
☙ to nourish Blood and invigorate Blood circulation
☙ moistens the Intestines and moves stool

USES
Dang Gui is a gynecological tonic, ideal for deficient Blood syndromes that may lead to menstrual irregularities. It can relieve pain from stagnant Blood, and is used with *Huang Qi* and fresh ginger in traditional stews made to relieve postpartum pains. As a laxative, it is especially helpful for the elderly.

DANG SHEN

PARTS USED
Root
TASTE
Sweet
CHARACTER
Neutral
BOTANICAL NAME
Codonopsis pilosula
COMMON NAME
Codonopsis, tang-shen, asiabell root
MERIDIANS
Spleen, Lung

Dang Shen is often used as an alternative to Korean ginseng (*Ren Shen*). It is considered gentler and more yin and is traditionally taken by nursing mothers. It is a popular ingredient of "Change of Season Soup" (which also contains *Huang Qi*, *Shan Yao*, and *Gou Qi Zi*).

ACTIONS
Blood tonic (increases red blood cells), hypotensive, immune stimulant, nervous stimulant, raises blood sugar levels

INDICATIONS
☙ to invigorate Spleen, Stomach, and Middle *Jiao*
☙ to replenish Spleen, and Lung *Qi*
☙ to nourish Body Fluids

USES
Dang Shen is an important *Qi* tonic. It is ideal for deficiency ailments characterized by tiredness, loss of appetite, aching limbs, palpitations, chronic coughs, and shortness of breath. It is traditionally used for deficient *Wei Qi* in soups and stews, and also helps Body Fluids.

DU HUO

PARTS USED
Root
TASTE
Pungent, bitter
CHARACTER
Slightly warm
BOTANICAL NAME
Angelica pubescens
COMMON NAME
Pubescent angelica
MERIDIANS
Kidney, Urinary Bladder

Du Hou is used to combat attack by the external pathogens Wind and Damp, so is helpful for superficial syndromes including colds and rheumatism or *Bi* syndrome (arthritis). It is the main ingredient in *Du Huo Ji Sheng Tang*, which is used for arthritis and back pain.

ACTIONS
antirheumatic, analgesic, anti-inflammatory, sedative, hypotensive, nervous stimulant

INDICATIONS
☙ to dispel Wind and Damp

USES
Du Huo is especially used for Wind–Damp problems affecting the lower back and legs, as well as for headaches and toothache. It is combined with *Fang Feng* for leg pains, and with *Ma Huang* for Wind–Cold where there are generalized aches and pains but no obvious fever. It is used with *Gao Ben* for headaches.

CONTRAINDICATIONS
Avoid in pregnancy, in cases of diarrhea or abdominal fullness.

CONTRAINDICATIONS
Avoid in attack by external evils.

CONTRAINDICATIONS
Avoid in yin deficiency and excess Fire symptoms.

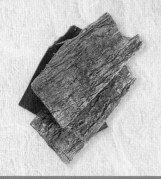
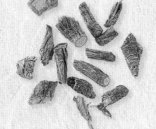
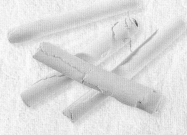

DU ZHONG

PARTS USED
Bark
TASTE
Sweet
CHARACTER
Warm
MERIDIANS
Liver, Kidney

BOTANICAL NAME
Eucommia ulmoides
COMMON NAME
Eucommia

Du Zhong was listed in Shen Nong's herbal and is an important yang tonic. The tree is the only surviving member of its genus and was first collected by Western plant hunters in the 1880s. Extracts have been used to treat high blood pressure.

ACTIONS
diuretic, hypotensive, reduces cholesterol levels, sedative, uterine relaxant

INDICATIONS
◉ tonifies Liver and Kidney *Qi*
◉ smoothes the flow of *Qi* and Blood to strengthen bones and muscles
◉ pacifies the fetus

USES
Du Zhong is used for Kidney weakness, characterized by low back pain, frequent urination, impotence, and weakness in the lower part of the body, and is associated with threatened miscarriage. It is often combined with *Bu Gu Zhi* for deficient Kidney yang or with *Gui Zhi* and *Du Huo* for problems associated with Cold–Damp.

FANG FENG

PART USED
Root
TASTE
Pungent, sweet
CHARACTER
Slightly warm
MERIDIANS
Liver, Spleen, Urinary Bladder

BOTANICAL NAME
Ledebouriella sesloides
COMMON NAME
Siler

The literal meaning of *Fang Feng* is "guard against wind," and the herb was a favorite for combating the ills which the Chinese believed blew in with the powerful winds from central Asia. It has been used medicinally for at least two thousand years and is also effective as an antidote to arsenic.

ACTIONS
antispasmodic, antibacterial, antifungal, febrifuge

INDICATIONS
◉ to disperse Wind evil and relieve exterior syndromes
◉ to clear Damp

USES
Fang Feng is used for both Wind–Heat and Wind–Cold syndromes, with symptoms of feverish chills, headache, and body pains, as in colds and flu. It is also used for certain types of arthritis (*Bi* syndrome), involving Wind and Cold symptoms, and for irritant skin rashes.

FU LING

PARTS USED
Sclerotium of the fungus found on pine tree roots
TASTE
Sweet, neutral
CHARACTER
Neutral
MERIDIANS
Lung, Spleen, Heart, Urinary Bladder

BOTANICAL NAME
Wolfiporia cocos
COMMON NAME
Tuckahoe, Indian bread, China root

Fu Ling is one of the many fungi used in Chinese medicine. As well as the main body of the fungus, the brown skin (*Fu Ling Pi*) is used as a diuretic, and the central part of the sclerotium is sometimes separated as *Fu Shen* and used as a strong calming remedy for the Heart.

ACTIONS
diuretic, sedative, hypoglycemic

INDICATIONS
◉ clears Dampness and regulates Water metabolism
◉ strengthens the Spleen, Stomach and Middle *Jiao*; transforms Phlegm
◉ to calm the Heart and *Shen* (spirit)

USES
As an effective diuretic, *Fu Ling* is used for such problems as scanty urination, edema, or painful urinary dysfunction – often with *Ze Xie* and *Gui Zhi*. As a calming Heart remedy, it is useful for palpitations and insomnia, and is used with *Chen Pi* and other herbs where Phlegm and Body Fluid problems lead to abdominal bloating.

CONTRAINDICATIONS
Avoid in deficient yin and active Fire symptoms.

CONTRAINDICATIONS
Avoid if headaches are associated with deficient yin.

CONTRAINDICATIONS
Avoid in cases involving excessive urination or prolapse of the urogenital organs.

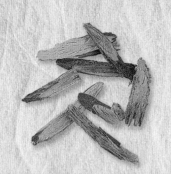
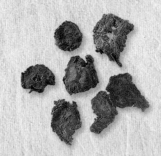

GAN GAO

BOTANICAL NAME
Glycyrrhiza uralensis
COMMON NAME
Licorice

PARTS USED
Root
TASTE
Sweet
CHARACTER
Neutral
MERIDIANS
Heart, Lung, Spleen, Stomach

One of China's most important tonic herbs, *Gan Cao* is described by Shen Nong as "sweet and balanced to treat the five *Zang* organs, six *Fu* organs, cold and heat, and evil *Qi*," adding that taking plenty of it could prolong life.

ACTIONS
antibacterial, anti-inflammatory, antispasmodic, antiallergenic, antitussive, hypotensive, steroidal action, cholagogue

INDICATIONS
☺ invigorates *Qi* function
☺ clears Heat and detoxifies Fire poisons
☺ moistens the Lung and stops coughing
☺ soothes spasms and relieves pain
☺ moderates the function of other herbs

USES
Gan Cao is used for problems of *Qi* deficiency – it is combined with *Dang Shen*, for example, if the problem is to do with Spleen *Qi*, or with *Gui Zhi* to nourish the Heart. It is used for coughs and asthma, and in Damp and Fire problems, e.g., boils, abscesses, or rashes.

GAO BEN

BOTANICAL NAME
Ligusticum sinense
COMMON NAME
Chinese lovage, straw weed

PARTS USED
Root and rhizome
TASTE
Pungent
CHARACTER
Warm
MERIDIANS
Urinary Bladder

Closely related to the lovage (*Ligusticum levisticum* syn. *Levisticum officinale*) used as a culinary seasoning in the West, *Gao Ben* is widely used, according to Chinese folk tradition, for menstrual problems and after childbirth, although its main medicinal uses are for chills and pain relief.

ACTIONS
antifungal, analgesic, antispasmodic

INDICATIONS
☺ to clear Wind–Cold symptoms
☺ to clear Wind–Damp symptoms

USES
Gao Ben is used for various types of headaches, migraine, joint pain, toothache, and arthritis, which can be associated with Wind, Cold, or Damp syndromes.

GE GEN

BOTANICAL NAME
Pueraria lobata
COMMON NAME
Kudzu vine

PART USED
Root
TASTE
Sweet, pungent
CHARACTER
Cool
MERIDIANS
Spleen, Stomach

Ge Gen has been condemned as a pernicious weed in the USA. Since its introduction from Japan in 1876, the plant has been described as a "vegetative plague" in southern forests and fields. Research has highlighted its use in combating alcoholism.

ACTIONS
antispasmodic, circulatory stimulant, febrifuge, mild hypotensive, reduces blood sugar

INDICATIONS
☺ to disperse Wind, Heat and Cold evils
☺ to raise the yang *Qi*
☺ to relieve skin eruptions, produce Body Fluids and cool the body

USES
Ge Gen is traditionally given for feverish chills and in the early stages of measles with other herbs. It raises yang *Qi*, so it is also used to combat diarrhea and dysentery associated with Damp Heat; to relieve symptoms of raised blood pressure, headaches and dizziness; and can help in coronary heart disease.

CONTRAINDICATIONS
Avoid in *Shi* syndrome (abdominal fullness).

CONTRAINDICATIONS
Avoid where there is internal Heat due to yin deficiency.

CONTRAINDICATIONS
Avoid in cases of stomach chills and if there is excessive sweating.

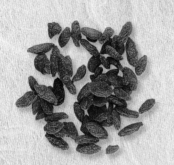

GOU QI ZI

PARTS USED
Fruit
TASTE
Sweet
CHARACTER
Neutral
MERIDIANS
Liver, Kidney

BOTANICAL NAME
Lycium barbarum
COMMON NAME
*Wolfberry,
matrimony vine*

Both fruits and root bark (*Di Gu Pi*) are used in Chinese medicine – the root bark is listed among Shen Nong's "superior woods" as a remedy for "evil *Qi*." The fruits are a more common remedy, used in a traditional tonic wine and combined with *Wu Wei Zi* for general debility.

ACTIONS
hypotensive, hypoglycemic, immune stimulant, Liver tonic and restorative, lowers blood cholesterol levels

INDICATIONS
☻ to nourish Liver and Kidney yin
☻ to nourish the Blood
☻ to brighten the eyes

USES
A restorative congee (*see* page 110) is made using the berries. This is used for Kidney *Qi* deficiency, typified by impotence, low back pain, dizziness and tinnitus. The berries are also combined with *Ju Hua* as a remedy for Liver deficiency and are used in washes for poor eyesight or eye strain.

GU YA

PARTS USED
Sprouted seeds
TASTE
Sweet
CHARACTER
Neutral
MERIDIANS
Spleen, Stomach

BOTANICAL NAME
Orzya sativa
COMMON NAME
Rice

As well as being China's staple food and used in therapeutic congee, various parts of the rice plant are also regarded as medicinal. The sprouted seeds are used to support a weak digestion, while the root (*Nuo Dao Gen*) is more focused on Lung, Liver, and Kidney meridians, and is used in low-grade fevers and to reduce sweating.

ACTIONS
Digestive tonic

INDICATIONS
☻ to improve digestion and appetite
☻ to remove food stagnation

USES
Sprouted rice seeds are used with *Chen Pi* and *Sha Ren* to stimulate appetite and clear food stagnation. Like sprouted barley (*Mai Ya*), sprouted rice is also believed to reduce milk flow at weaning.

GUI ZHI

PARTS USED
Twigs
TASTE
Pungent, sweet
CHARACTER
Warm
MERIDIANS
*Heart, Lung,
Urinary Bladder*

BOTANICAL NAME
Cinnamomum cassia
COMMON NAME
Cinnamon, cassia

Both the twigs and bark (*Rou Gui*) are used medicinally – the bark is considered to be much hotter and focused on Spleen, Kidney, Liver, and Urinary Bladder meridians. While *Gui Zhi* is seen as warming the exterior and channels, *Rou Gui* (like the tree's bark) is more central in its direction for warming the abdominal organs.

ACTIONS
antibacterial, antifungal, antiviral, analgesic, carminative, cardiotonic, diuretic

INDICATIONS
☻ to warm the channels and collaterals
☻ to disperse Cold
☻ to improve circulation of yang *Qi*
☻ to strengthen Heart yang

USES
Gui Zhi is a useful remedy for exterior Cold – as in common colds and arthritic problems associated with cold weather. It is also used for palpitations and shortness of breath, and is combined with *Fu Ling, Gan Cao,* or *Dan Shen* for various heart problems, including angina pectoris.

CONTRAINDICATIONS
Avoid in cases of excess Heat, and Spleen deficiency with Dampness.

CONTRAINDICATIONS
Not to be taken by nursing mothers or where there are no signs of food stagnation.

CONTRAINDICATIONS
Avoid in feverish conditions, excess Heat or Fire, and in pregnancy.

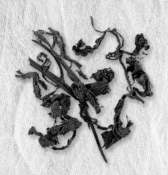
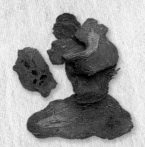
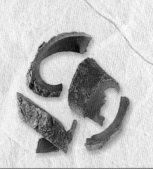

HAN LIAN CAO

PARTS USED
Aerial parts
TASTE
Sweet, sour
CHARACTER
Cold
MERIDIANS
Liver, Kidney

BOTANICAL NAME
Eclipta prostrata
COMMON NAME
False daisy

Han Lian Cao is one of the main herbs used to nourish yin. It is an important liver and spleen remedy in Ayurvedic medicine and is also used in oils to combat hair loss. In Chinese folk tradition, it is used for skin problems such as athlete's foot and dermatitis.

ACTIONS
antibacterial, hemostatic

INDICATION
◉ to nourish Liver and Kidney yin
◉ to clear Heat from the Blood and stop bleeding

USES
Han Lian Cao is one of the main tonics for Kidney and Liver yin; it can be combined with *Nu Zhen Zi* for severe deficiency syndromes, which may be characterized by blurred vision, tinnitus, prematurely graying hair and dizziness. As a styptic, it is combined with appropriate herbs to stop various types of bleeding – with *Ai Ye,* for example, for uterine bleeding.

HE SHOU WU

PARTS USED
Root
TASTE
Sweet, bitter, astringent
CHARACTER
Slightly warm
MERIDIANS
Liver, Kidney

BOTANICAL NAME
Polygonum multiflorum
COMMON NAME
Fleeceflower

He Shou Wu is also known in the West as *Fo Ti* from its Cantonese name. The root is the main part used, although fleeceflower stems (*Ye Jiao Teng*) are also used as a Heart and Liver tonic to calm the nerves and improve Blood circulation.

ACTIONS
antibacterial, cardiotonic, hormonal action, hyperglycemic, laxative, liver stimulant, reduces blood cholesterol

INDICATIONS
◉ to replenish Liver and Kidney *Jing* and nourish Blood
◉ to detoxify Fire poisons
◉ to clear exterior Wind
◉ to lubricate the Intestines (laxative)

USES
He Shou Wu is useful at the menopause to tonify Liver and Kidney and can help deficiencies here at any age. It is effective for constipation in the elderly and is used with such herbs as *Ren Shen* and *Dang Gui* for chronic debility. With *Xuan Shen* and *Lian Qiao*, it can relieve abscesses.

HOU PO

PARTS USED
Bark
TASTE
Pungent, bitter
CHARACTER
Warm
MERIDIAN
Spleen, Stomach, Lung, Large Intestine

BOTANICAL NAME
Magnolia officinalis
COMMON NAME
Magnolia

Magnolia bark, used since the days of Shen Nong, is classified as an aromatic herb to clear Dampness. The flowers, *Hou Po Hua,* are used in a similar way but are more focused on Dampness in the chest area than the lower abdomen.

ACTIONS
antibacterial, antifungal, carminative, hypotensive

INDICATIONS
◉ to move *Qi,* transform Dampness, and relieve food stagnation in the stomach
◉ to warm and transform Phlegm and invigorate Spleen *Qi*
◉ to reverse the upward flow of *Qi*

USES
Hou Po is mainly used for coughs and vomiting, which are both associated with Dampness and with dysfunction in *Qi* flow. It is combined with herbs like *Zhi Shi* and *Ban Xia* in cases of food stagnation or abdominal bloating, and with *Ma Huang* and *Xing Ren* for clearing productive coughs.

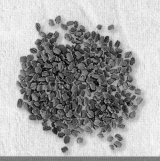
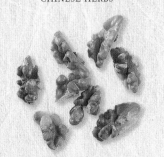
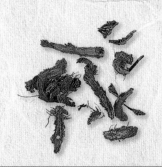

HU LA BA

BOTANICAL NAME
Trigonella foenum-graecum
COMMON NAME
Fenugreek

PARTS USED
Seeds
TASTE
Pungent, bitter
CHARACTER
Very warm
MERIDIANS
Kidney

Fenugreek is a popular culinary herb, familiar from Middle Eastern and Oriental cookery. It is a very warming remedy, ideal for all sorts of colds and chills affecting the abdomen. In the Middle East, the plant is known as "*hilba*" – very similar in pronunciation to its Chinese name – and is used for menstrual pain and colic.

ACTIONS
antiparasitic, laxative, galactagogue

INDICATIONS
☺ to warm the Kidneys and dispel Cold
☺ to relieve pain

USES
Hu Lu Ba is mainly used for pains in the abdomen and groin where there is Kidney weakness. It can be combined with fennel seeds (*Xiao Hui Xiang*) for hernia-like disorders, as well as for period pains and with other Kidney herbs, such as *Bu Gu Zhi,* for pain and cold in the lower abdomen and back.

HU TAO REN

BOTANICAL NAME
Juglans regia
COMMON NAME
Walnut

PARTS USED:
Seed (nut kernel)
TASTE
Sweet
CHARACTER
Warm
MERIDIANS
Lung, Kidney, Large Intestine

In the West, walnuts are valued as a gentle nutrient and digestive remedy while their oil is a good source of essential fatty acids. In China, the nuts are regarded more as a yang tonic, especially helpful for the kidneys.

ACTIONS
astringent, laxative, anti-inflammatory, mild hypoglycemic, nutrient (encourages weight gain), dissolves urinary stones

INDICATIONS
☺ to reinforce Kidney yang and strengthen the back
☺ to warm and strengthen Lung *Qi*
☺ to moisten the Intestines (laxative)

USES
Hu Tao Ren is used for symptoms of Kidney deficiency – typically low back pain and urinary dysfunction. It is valuable for constipation in the elderly (often in combination with *Huo Ma Ren* and other herbs), and it is combined with *Ren Shen* for Lung deficiency problems.

HUANG LIAN

BOTANICAL NAME
Coptis chinensis
COMMON NAME
Chinese gold thread

PARTS USED
Root and rhizome
TASTE
Bitter
CHARACTER
Cold
MERIDIANS
Heart, Liver, Stomach, Large Intestine

Huang Lian is a very cold herb which will clear almost any sort of Heat problem. Shen Nong referred to it as *Wang Lian* (king lily), and listed the plant among the "superior" herbs, suggesting that regular use of the plant would also improve the memory.

ACTIONS
antibacterial, hypotensive, stimulates acetylcholine production, sedative, anti-inflammatory, antifungal, cholagogue

INDICATIONS
☺ to clear Heat, Fire, Fire poisons and Damp Heat
☺ to calm Heart Fire
☺ to drain Stomach Fire

USES
Huang Lian is taken for many sorts of Heat-related problems, including infections and inflammations. It is used for gastroenteritis, food poisoning, fevers, conjunctivitis, boils, abscesses, and mouth inflammations. As it calms Heart Fire, the herb is also used for palpitations, insomnia, and irritability.

CONTRAINDICATIONS
Avoid in pregnancy, if there are Fire symptoms, or in deficient yin.

CONTRAINDICATIONS
Avoid in cases involving Heat, Phlegm, or Fire symptoms and deficient yin.

CONTRAINDICATIONS
Avoid if there is diarrhea, *Jing* deficiency, or Cold Deficient Stomach.

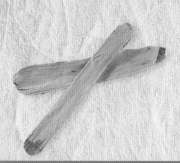
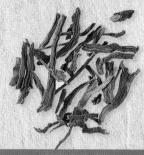
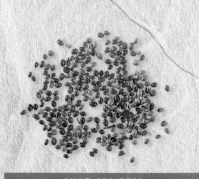

HUANG QI

PARTS USED
Root
TASTE
Sweet
CHARACTER
Slightly warm
MERIDIANS
Spleen, Lung

BOTANICAL NAME
Astragalus membranaceus
COMMON NAME
Milk vetch

Huang Qi is an important Qi tonic for younger people (*Ren Shen* was considered better for people over 40). The two herbs are often used together as a general tonic. *Huang Qi* is an important immune stimulant.

ACTIONS
antispasmodic, diuretic, cholagogue, antibacterial, hypoglycemic, nervous stimulant, hypotensive, immune stimulant

INDICATIONS
- tonifies *Qi* and Blood
- stabilizes *Wei Qi* and stops sweating
- clears pus; accelerates wound healing
- regulates Water metabolism and clears edema

USES
Huang Qi is used for deficient Spleen syndromes causing as poor appetite, tiredness, and diarrhea, and for weakened *Wei Qi*, which may manifest as recurrent infections or respiratory problems. It is added to remedies for fluid retention and chronic sores, and is given after childbirth to help restore *Qi* and Blood.

CONTRAINDICATIONS
Avoid in excess (*Shi*) syndromes or if there is deficient yin.

HUANG QIN

PARTS USED
Root
TASTE
Bitter
CHARACTER
Cold
MERIDIANS
Lung, Heart, Gall Bladder, Stomach, Large Intestine

BOTANICAL NAME
Scutellaria baicalensis
COMMON NAME
Baikal skullcap

Western varieties of skullcap are classified as nervines or sedatives, but the Chinese member of the family is primarily used for clearing Damp Heat – both external and internal.

ACTIONS
antibacterial, antispasmodic, diuretic, febrifuge, lowers blood cholesterol

INDICATIONS
- to clear Heat and quell Fire
- to drain Damp Heat
- to calm the fetus (in threatened miscarriage)
- to eliminate heat in the Lungs and calm Liver yang

USES
Huang Qin is used with other cooling herbs like *Huang Lian* for feverish chills with symptoms of thick yellow sputum, thirst, and irritability. Internal Damp–Heat problems generally manifest as dysentery-like disorders, and the herb is used for gastroenteritis and diarrhea, as well as urinary tract infections.

CONTRAINDICATIONS
Not to be used for a person without true Heat and Dampness symptoms.

HUO MA REN

PARTS USED
Seeds
TASTE
Sweet
CHARACTER
Neutral
MERIDIANS
Spleen, Stomach, Large Intestine

BOTANICAL NAME
Cannabis sativa
COMMON NAME
Cannabis, hemp, marijuana

Although cannabis is generally regarded as a recreational drug, it is also an important medicinal plant. In the West, it is used – legislation permitting – as an anti-emetic and to relieve symptoms of muscular sclerosis. In China, the seeds are considered primarily as a gentle and moist laxative.

ACTIONS
laxative, hypotensive

INDICATIONS
- to lubricate the Intestines
- to nourish yin
- to clear Heat and heal sores

USES
Huo Ma Ren is a specific for constipation in the elderly, often related to lack of energy and Body Fluids. It is combined with *Dang Gui* or made into *Ma Zi Ren Wan* (cannabis seed pills), which also contain *Da Huang*, *Bai Shao*, *Xing Ren*, *Hou Po*, and *Zhi Shi*.

CONTRAINDICATIONS
Not to be used in cases of diarrhea.

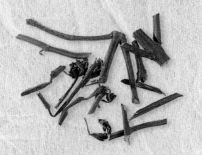
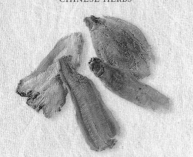
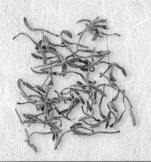

HUO XIANG

PARTS USE
Aerial parts
TASTE
Pungent
CHARACTER
Slightly warm
MERIDIANS
Lung, Spleen, Stomach

BOTANICAL NAME
Pogostemon cablin
COMMON NAME
Patchouli

Many Chinese medicinal herb names actually represent more than one species and *Huo Xiang* can just as easily be *Agastache rugosa* (giant wrinkled hyssop). The herb – of whichever species – is categorized as an aromatic to clear Damp.

ACTIONS
antibacterial, antifungal, diaphoretic, digestive tonic

INDICATIONS
☺ to transform Dampness in Spleen and Stomach
☺ to harmonize the Middle *Jiao* and combat nausea
☺ to dispel cold

USES
Huo Xiang is used for a range of Damp problems – from common colds to morning sickness in pregnancy. This herb is very aromatic and good for clearing catarrh (often combined with *Zu Su Ye*). For abdominal distension, it is used with *Ban Xia*.

JIE GENG

PARTS USED
Root
TASTE
Pungent, bitter
CHARACTER
Neutral
MERIDIANS
Lung

BOTANICAL NAME
Platycodon grandiflorum
COMMON NAME
Balloon flower

Balloon flowers are grown as a garden ornamental in the West. Their striking blue or white flowers appear as a large balloon before opening out fully. This herb has been used as a cough remedy since the days of Shen Nong.

ACTIONS
antibacterial, expectorant, hypoglycemic, reduces blood cholesterol levels

INDICATIONS
☺ to circulate Lung *Qi*
☺ to expel Phlegm caused by Wind–Cold and Wind–Heat
☺ to direct other herbs upward
☺ to clear pus in Lung or throat abscesses

USES
Jie Geng is a good expectorant for productive coughs with profuse Phlegm associated with infections. It can be combined with *Sang Ye, Ju Hua, Bo He,* and *Gan Cao* in *Sang Ju Yin,* which is a remedy given for coughs and colds. *Jie Geng* is also helpful for sore throats and hoarseness.

JIN YIN HUA

PARTS USED
Flowers
TASTE
Sweet
CHARACTER
Cold
MERIDIANS
Lung, Stomach, Large Intestine

BOTANICAL NAME
Lonicera japonica
COMMON NAME
Honeysuckle

The Chinese honeysuckle is regarded in the West as a popular garden climber with a rich scent, rather than as a medicinal herb. The flowers and stems (*Jin Yin Teng*) have been used to treat feverish colds since at least the seventh century.

ACTIONS
antibacterial, antiviral, hypotensive

INDICATIONS
☺ to clear Heat and Fire Poisons
☺ to clear Damp Heat in the lower burner
☺ to expel external Wind–Heat

USES
Jin Yin Hua is used for feverish colds caused by Wind and Heat. It is also effective for internal Heat problems characterized by dysentery-like symptoms or urinary infections. As it clears Fire Poisons, it is also used for boils and abscesses.

CONTRAINDICATIONS
Avoid in fevers and interior Heat syndromes.

CONTRAINDICATIONS
Avoid in cases of tuberculosis.

CONTRAINDICATIONS
Avoid in deficient and Cold conditions.

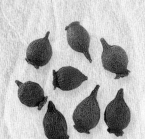
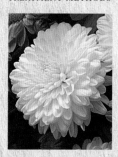

JIN YING ZI

PARTS USED
Fruit (hips)
TASTE
Sweet, astringent
CHARACTER
Neutral
MERIDIANS
Kidney, Urinary Bladder, Large Intestine

BOTANICAL NAME
Rosa laevigata
COMMON NAME
Cherokee rose

Both Cherokee rosehips and Japanese rosebuds (*Mei Gui Hua – R. rugosa*) are used in Chinese medicine, although their actions are quite different. *Mei Gui Hua* is regarded more as a *Qi* and Blood tonic for the Liver, while *Jin Ying Zi* is focused on the Kidney and *Jing*.

ACTIONS
astringent, antibacterial, antiviral, reduces cholesterol levels, tonifies uterus

INDICATIONS
☙ to consolidate Kidney *Qi* and retain *Jing*
☙ to restrain leakage from the Intestines

USES
Like all members of the rose family, *Jin Ying Zi* is very astringent – so is a good antidiarrheal. It is associated with the Kidneys, so is used for treating urinary problems, as well as impotence and premature ejaculation. It is combined with herbs like *Dang Shen*, *Shan Yao*, and *Bai Zhu* for diarrhea associated with deficient spleen.

JU HUA

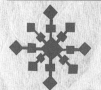

PARTS USED
Flowers
TASTE
Pungent, sweet, bitter
CHARACTER
Cool
MERIDIANS
Lung, Liver

BOTANICAL NAME
Dendranthema x grandiflorum
COMMON NAME
Chrysanthemum

*J*u Hua are the flowerheads of the familiar florist's chrysanthemums, which make a popular cooling tea in China – readily available in cartons from takeaways and supermarkets. The herb was listed by Shen Nong and has been used for at least two thousand years.

ACTIONS
antibacterial, antifungal, antiviral, anti-inflammatory, hypotensive, peripheral vasodilator

INDICATIONS
☙ to disperse Wind and Heat
☙ to clear Liver Heat and calm Liver Wind
☙ to neutralize toxins

USES
Ascending Liver yang or Wind–Heat in the Liver channel are associated with sore, red eyes, dizziness, and headaches. As *Ju Hua* is good in both conditions, it is said to "brighten the eyes" and is used for colds or feverish conditions where bloodshot eyes are a key characteristic. It also reduces high blood pressure.

KUAN DONG HUA

PARTS USED
Flower bud
TASTE
Pungent
CHARACTER
Warm
MERIDIANS
Lung

BOTANICAL NAME
Tussilago farfara
COMMON NAME
Coltsfoot

In the West, both leaves and flowers of coltsfoot are used for coughs as an expectorant. The Chinese have used the plant in much the same way since the days of Shen Nong. Its Chinese name means "welcome winter flower" – as in Europe it is one of the earliest spring blooms, with the flowers opening before the leaves appear.

ACTIONS
Relaxing expectorant, anticatarrhal, demulcent. Topically used as a tissue healer and demulcent

INDICATIONS
☙ to moisten the Lung and send *Qi* downward

USES
Kuan Dong Hua is, as in the West, used for a range of coughs and wheezing, including chronic bronchitis, asthma, and whooping cough. They are specific for coughs with profuse or blood-streaked phlegm, and are combined with herbs like *Xing Ren*, *Wu Wei Zi*, and *Ban Xia*.

CONTRAINDICATIONS
Avoid in excess Fire and Heat syndromes.

CONTRAINDICATIONS
Avoid in cases of diarrhea and *Qi* deficiency.

CONTRAINDICATIONS
It contains pyrrolizidine alkaloids (linked with liver cancer) and is banned in some countries.

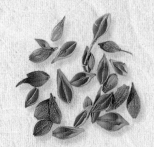
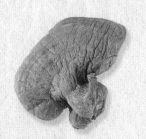

LIAN QIAO

BOTANICAL NAME
Forsythia suspensa
COMMON NAME
Forsythia

PARTS USED
Fruit
TASTE
Bitter
CHARACTER
Slightly cold
MERIDIANS
Lung, Heart, Gall Bladder

Forsythia is familiar in the West as a yellow-flowered garden shrub (brought to Europe in 1844 by the Scottish explorer Robert Fortune and named after the Scottish botanist William Forsyth). The herb is listed by Shen Nong and it is often used with *Jin Yin Hua*, as the two seem to work better in combination.

ACTIONS
antibacterial, antiemetic, antiparasitic

INDICATIONS
◉ to clear Heat and Fire poisons
◉ to expel Wind–Heat
◉ to dissipate nodules and swellings

USES
Lian Qiao is an effective herb for clearing any infection or abscess. It is traditionally used for feverish colds that are characterized by sore throats and headaches, for infections – involving swollen neck glands or lymph nodes – and for urinary tract infections. It is used with *Chi Shao* and *Ma Huang* in skin eruptions.

CONTRAINDICATIONS
Avoid in cases of diarrhea linked to deficient Spleen, fevers linked to deficient *Qi,* and purulent abscesses.

LING ZHI

BOTANICAL NAME
Ganoderma lucidem
COMMON NAME
Reishi mushroom

PARTS USED
Fruiting body
TASTE
Sweet
CHARACTER
Slightly warm
MERIDIANS
Lung, Heart, Spleen, Liver, Kidney

The reishi mushroom was highly regarded by the Taoists as a spiritual tonic which they believed could enhance longevity. It was as "shaman's fungus" and was thought to be especially good for Heart *Qi*.

ACTIONS
antiviral, immune stimulant, expectorant, antitussive, antihistamine, antitumor, reduces blood pressure and cholesterol levels

INDICATIONS
◉ to tonify *Qi* and Blood
◉ to calm the Heart and Shen

USES
Ling Zhi is traditionally used for general debility, lung problems (including asthma and chronic bronchitis), and for problems related to Heart disharmonies, such as insomnia, palpitations, forgetfulness, and hypertension. It is now known to stimulate the immune system and has been used for chronic fatigue syndrome and AIDS.

CONTRAINDICATIONS
Do not take if there are no signs of weakness or deficiency.

LONG DAN CAO

BOTANICAL NAME
Gentiana scabra
COMMON NAME
Chinese gentian

PARTS USED
Root and rhizome
TASTE
Bitter
CHARACTER
Cold
MERIDIANS
Liver, Gall Bladder, Stomach

Shen Nong lists *Long Dan Cao* among the "superior herbs," recommending it for treating "Cold and Heat in the bones and evil *Qi*." It is mainly used as a Liver remedy for jaundice and related problems.

ACTIONS
antibacterial, anti-inflammatory, digestive and appetite stimulant, hyperglycemic

INDICATIONS
◉ to eliminate Heat and Dampness from Liver and Gall Bladder
◉ to pacify Liver Fire

USES
Long Dan Cao is used with herbs like *Huang Qin* and *Chai Hu* to calm Liver Fire, which is typified by red swollen eyes and ears, sore throat, or symptoms of jaundice. It is used for other "hot" conditions, including skin irritations, acute urinary infections, and high blood pressure associated with dizziness.

CONTRAINDICATIONS
Avoid if there are no symptoms of Heat, Fire or Dampness.

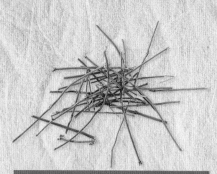

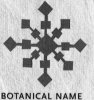

MA HUANG

PARTS USED
Twigs or stems
TASTE
Pungent, slightly bitter
CHARACTER
Warm
MERIDIANS
Lung, Urinary Bladder

BOTANICAL NAME
Ephedra sinica
COMMON NAME
Ephedra

Ma Huang is the original source of the drug ephedrine, which is used for asthmatic and catarrhal conditions. The plant was included in Shen Nong's herbal and is mainly used for external or superficial problems, especially Wind–Cold. The root (*Ma Huang Gen*) is an astringent.

ACTIONS
antispasmodic, antibacterial, antiviral, diaphoretic, diuretic, febrifuge

INDICATIONS
☻ for excessive superficial syndromes due to Wind–Cold
☻ to encourage sweating
☻ to mobilize Lung *Qi*
☻ to increase urination

USES
Ma Huang is used for chills and fevers associated with attack by external Cold or Wind. It works well with *Gui Zhi*, as the two herbs seem to enhance each other's action. The herb is given for asthma and breathing difficulties associated with Lung *Qi* stagnation.

MI MENG HUA

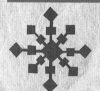

PARTS USED
Flower
TASTE
Sweet
CHARACTER
Cool
MERIDIAN
Liver

BOTANICAL NAME
Buddleia officinalis
COMMON NAME
Buddleia

Another of the garden ornamentals introduced to Europe by the 19th-century plant hunters, buddleia is used mainly – via its emphasis on the Liver meridian – for eye problems. Its use dates back to the Song Dynasty in the tenth century CE.

ACTIONS
antispasmodic, mild diuretic

INDICATIONS
☻ to clear Heat in the Liver
☻ to benefit the eyes

USES
Mi Meng Hua is used for numerous eye problems – from red, strained eyes to cataracts. The herb is combined with remedies like *Gou Qi Zi* for poor eyesight, such as cataracts, which can be related to deficient Liver and Kidney energy.

MU DAN PI

PARTS USED
Root bark
TASTE
Bitter, pungent
CHARACTER
Slightly cold
MERIDIANS
Heart, Liver, Kidney

BOTANICAL NAME
Paeonia suffruticosa
COMMON NAME
Tree peony, moutan peony

The tree peony – another popular garden ornamental in the West – is an important herb for cooling Blood. It was first listed in a 12th-century Chinese herbal known as the "Pouch of Pearls" (*Zhen Zhu Nang*).

ACTIONS
antibacterial, antiallergenic, anti-inflammatory, analgesic, hypotensive, sedative

INDICATIONS
☻ to clear Heat and cool the Blood
☻ to invigorate Blood and clear Blood stagnation
☻ to clear ascending Liver Fire

USES
Mu Dan Pi is used for problems like nosebleeds or blood in the sputum or vomit, which Chinese medicine associates with Heat in the Blood, often combined with *Chi Shao*. It is also used for menstrual problems (including period pain) linked to Blood stagnation, and for various internal inflammations.

CONTRAINDICATIONS
Avoid in deficiency syndromes or in cases of high blood pressure.

CONTRAINDICATIONS
None known.

CONTRAINDICATIONS
Avoid in pregnancy or in cases of diarrhea.

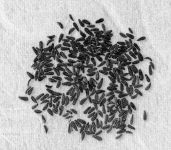

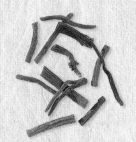

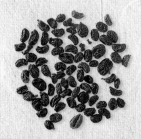

NIU BANG ZI

PARTS USED
Seeds
TASTE
Pungent, bitter
CHARACTER
Cold
MERIDIANS
Lung, Stomach

BOTANICAL NAME
Arctium lappa
COMMON NAME
Burdock

NIU XI

PARTS USED
Root
TASTE
Bitter, sour
CHARACTER
Neutral
MERIDIANS
Liver, Kidney

BOTANICAL NAME
Achyranthis bidentata
COMMON NAME
Two-toothed amaranthus

NU ZHEN ZI

PARTS USED
Berries
TASTE
Sweet, bitter
CHARACTER
Neutral
MERIDIANS
Liver, Kidney

BOTANICAL NAME
Ligustrum lucidum
COMMON NAME
Glossy privet, wax-leaf privet

While burdock leaves and roots are used in Western herbal medicine, mainly as cleansing remedies in skin and arthritic conditions, the Chinese use only the seeds. *Niu Bang Zi* was first listed in an 11th-century herbal, and today it is often used for common colds

ACTIONS
antibacterial, antifungal, diuretic, hypoglycemic, hypotensive, purgative

INDICATIONS
- to dispel Wind and Heat in the exterior
- to detoxify Fire poisons
- to encourage skin eruptions, such as measles
- to moisten the Intestines

USES
Niu Bang Zi is used for a variety of infectious conditions, including common colds, throat inflammations, tonsillitis, mumps, measles, abscesses, and carbuncles. It is often combined with herbs like *Jie Geng*, *Jin Yin Hua*, *Lian Qiao*, and *Bo He*.

Niu Xi translates as "ox knees," which may be a description of its knobbled stems but also points to its use as a Liver remedy. The Liver is associated with tendons, and, as there are a great many tendons in the knees, aching knees can often suggest stagnating Liver problems.

ACTIONS
analgesic, diuretic, hypotensive

INDICATIONS
- to invigorate Blood circulation and clear stagnant Blood
- to strengthen sinews and bones by nourishing the Liver and Kidneys
- to clear Damp Heat in the Lower *Jiao*
- to descend the flow of Blood and *Qi*

USES
As a Blood and Liver remedy, *Niu Xi* is included in remedies for menstrual problems. It is more commonly used for pains in the back and lower limbs, when it is often combined with *Du Zhong*. It is a directional remedy and helps to focus attention on the lower part of the body.

Nu Zhen Zi is one of the more important herbs for nourishing the Liver and Kidneys, and has been used since Shen Nong's days. *Nu Zhen* means "female chastity," a name that is based on its pale green/white evergreen leaves.

ACTIONS
antibacterial, cardiotonic, diuretic, immune stimulant

INDICATIONS
- to replenish and nourish deficient Liver and Kidney yin

USE
As a Liver and Kidney restorative, it will also darken prematurely graying hair and help improve the eyesight. It is included in various menopausal remedies and used with herbs like *Bu Gu Zhi* for lower back pains associated with Kidney weakness.

CONTRAINDICATIONS
Avoid in cases of diarrhea.

CONTRAINDICATIONS
Avoid in pregnancy and cases of menorrhagia.

CONTRAINDICATIONS
Avoid in diarrhea with deficiency of yang.

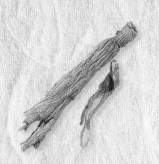
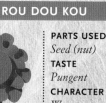
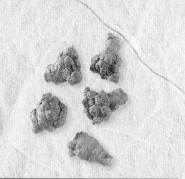

REN SHEN

PARTS USE
Root
TASTE
Sweet, slightly bitter
CHARACTER
Warm
MERIDIANS
Spleen, Lung, Heart

BOTANICAL NAME
Panax ginseng
COMMON NAME
Korean ginseng

Ginseng is China's most important *Qi* tonic, and has been used for over 5,000 years. It has been well researched and is known to be rich in compounds similar to human sex hormones – hence its reputation as an aphrodisiac.

ACTIONS
tonic, stimulant, reduces blood sugar and cholesterol levels, immunostimulant

INDICATIONS
◉ to replenish *Qi*
◉ to tonify the Spleen and Lungs
◉ to generate Body Fluids
◉ to benefit Heart *Qi* and calm *Shen*

USES
Ren Shen is a powerful, all-round tonic helping the body adapt to stressful situations, restore energy, and combat chronic weaknesses. It is good for the elderly and to strengthen the lungs. It is ideally taken for a month in late fall when the weather is changing from hot summer to cold winter and the body needs to adapt to a new environment.

CONTRAINDICATIONS
Avoid in Heat and deficient yin conditions.

ROU DOU KOU

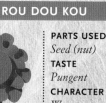

PARTS USED
Seed (nut)
TASTE
Pungent
CHARACTER
Warm
MERIDIANS
Spleen, Stomach, Large Intestine

BOTANICAL NAME
Myristica fragrans
COMMON NAME
Nutmeg

Nutmeg is familiar in the West as a kitchen seasoning, although it is a very potent herb which can cause delirium in high doses. The Chinese use it as a digestive remedy for the Spleen and Stomach.

ACTIONS
antispasmodic, antiemetic, appetite stimulant, anti-inflammatory, carminative, digestive stimulant

INDICATIONS
◉ to restrain leakage from the Intestines and stop diarrhea
◉ to warm the Spleen, Stomach, and Middle *Jiao*, and regulate *Qi* flow

USE
Rou Dou Kou is used largely for chronic diarrhea (including the "cock crow" variety associated with Kidney deficiency, when it is used with *Bu Gu Zhi, Da Zao, Sheng Jiang*, and other herbs in *Si Shen Wan* – pills of four miraculous drugs). It is also helpful for nausea, abdominal bloating, indigestion, and colic.

CONTRAINDICATIONS
Avoid in pregnancy, or in diarrhea caused by Heat factors. Large doses (over 5g) can produce convulsions.

SAN QI

PARTS USED
Root
TASTE
Sweet, slightly bitter
CHARACTER
Warm
MERIDIANS
Liver, Stomach

BOTANICAL NAME
Panax pseudoginseng
COMMON NAME
Notoginseng, pseudoginseng

San Qi (also known as *Tian Qi*) is a close relative of Korean ginseng, although it is mainly used to stop bleeding rather than as a *Qi* tonic. The plant was first listed by Li Shi Zhen in his 16th-century herbal, **Ben Cao Gang Mu.**

ACTIONS
antibacterial, anti-inflammatory, cardiotonic, circulator stimulant, diuretic, hemostatic, lowers blood sugar levels, peripheral vasodilator

INDICATIONS
◉ to stop bleeding and clear Blood stagnation
◉ to reduce swelling and relieve pain

USES
San Qi is used to clear any sort of blood clot or bleeding – such as swellings associated with traumatic wounds, soft tissue injuries, and bleeding. It is used in angina pectoris as well as in nosebleeds, abnormal uterine bleeding, and bleeding from gastric ulcers.

CONTRAINDICATION
Not to be used in pregnancy and with caution in deficient Blood syndromes.

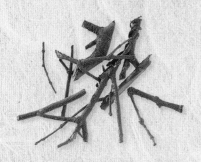
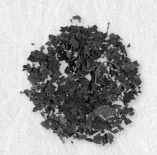
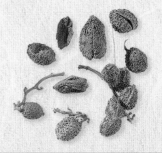

SANG JI SHENG

PARTS USED
Leaf stems
TASTE
Bitter
CHARACTER
Neutral
MERIDIANS
Liver, Kidney

BOTANICAL NAME
Loranthus parasiticus
COMMON NAME
Mulberry mistletoe

*S*ang Ji Sheng is derived from a parasitic plant, rather like mistletoe, which grows on mulberry trees. It was originally listed in the delightfully named "Grandfather Lei's Discussion of Herb Preparations" which dates from 470 CE.

ACTIONS
antiviral, cardiotonic, diuretic, hypotensive, sedative

INDICATIONS
☻ to tonify Liver and Kidney *Qi*
☻ to clear Wind, Cold and Damp
☻ to nourish Blood
☻ to strengthen sinews and bones

USES
Sang Ji Sheng can be used for *Bi* syndrome (arthritis) associated with Wind and Damp. It is combined with *Niu Xi* to focus the plant on the lower limbs and lower back in *Du Huo Ji Sheng Tang* (*see* pages 48–49). It is also used for high blood pressure and Heart problems associated with deficient Liver and Kidney yin.

SANG YE

PARTS USED
Leaves
TASTE
Sweet, bitter
CHARACTER
Cold
MERIDIANS
Lung, Liver

BOTANICAL NAME
Morus alba
COMMON NAME
Mulberry

*T*he mulberry is one of China's most versatile medicinal trees with leaves, root bark (*Sang Bai Pi*), fruit spikes (*Sang Shen*), and branches (*Sang Zhi*), all used in different ways.

ACTIONS
Various parts of the mulberry have been found to be analgesic, anti-asthmatic, antibacterial, antitussive, diaphoretic, diuretic, expectorant, hypotensive, sedative, and to reduce blood sugar levels

INDICATIONS
Leaves: ☻ to clear Wind and Heat
☻ to clear Heat in the Liver and Blood
Bark: ☻ to relieve coughing and clear Heat in the Lungs
☻ to reduce edema and promote urination

USES
Sang Ye is generally included in remedies for feverish colds, while *Sang Bai Pi* is a good cough remedy for hot conditions and asthma. *Sang Zhi* is mainly used for rheumatic pains, while *Sang Shen* is a yin tonic used to nourish the Blood that is helpful in cases of anemia.

SHA REN

PARTS USED
Fruit
TASTE
Pungent
CHARACTER
Warm
MERIDIANS
Spleen, Stomach, Kidney

BOTANICAL NAME
Amomum xanthioides
COMMON NAME
Bastard cardamom, grains of paradise

*S*ha Ren literally means "sand seeds." The plant looks and grows rather like reeds in damp places. It is sometimes used as a substitute for true cardamom (*Elettaria cardamomum*) in cooking and has been used in Chinese medicine since at least the fourteenth century.

ACTIONS
antiemetic

INDICATIONS
☻ to transform Dampness
☻ to warm the Spleen and Stomach and move *Qi*
☻ to calm the fetus

USES
Although little researched, *Sha Ren* is used in a number of prescriptions for digestive problems associated with stagnant *Qi*. It combats nausea and is used in pregnancy – both for morning sickness and, with *Sang Ji Sheng*, to help combat threatened miscarriage.

CONTRAINDICATIONS
Avoid in Heat syndromes.

CONTRAINDICATIONS
Avoid using *Sang Bai Pi* and *Sang Ye* for Cold conditions or *Sang Shen* for diarrhea.

CONTRAINDICATIONS
Avoid in deficient yin syndromes with Heat signs.

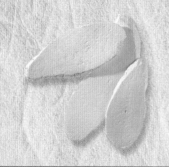
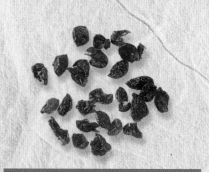

SHAN YAO

PARTS USED
Rhizome
TASTE
Sweet
CHARACTER
Neutral
MERIDIANS
Lung, Spleen, Kidney

BOTANICAL NAME
Dioscorea opposita
COMMON NAME
Chinese yam

Shan Yao is produced in the Henan Province near the Huai River, along with *Di Huang, Ju Hua*, and *Niu Xi*. It is sometimes called *Huai Shan*, just as *Niu Xi* is called *Huai Niu Xi*. It is one of the main herbs used to tonify *Qi*.

ACTIONS
antibacterial, cardiotonic, hypotensive, peripheral vasodilator, uterine stimulant

INDICATIONS
☻ to tonify Spleen and Stomach function
☻ to nourish the Lungs
☻ to strengthen the Kidneys and *Jing*

USES
Shan Yao is used in the main part as a digestive remedy for abdominal bloating, indigestion, and also for poor appetite that is associated with food stagnation.
Like its Western counterpart (*D. villosa*), it also has a hormonal action which has led to its use for postpartum pains and scanty periods.

SHAN ZHA

PARTS USED
Fruit
TASTE
Sour, sweet
CHARACTER
Slightly warm
MERIDIANS
Spleen, Stomach, Liver

BOTANICAL NAME
Crataegus pinnatifida
COMMON NAME
Chinese hawthorn

Hawthorn is used in the West, as a heart tonic and to normalize blood pressure. In contrast, the closely related Chinese species is seen as a digestive remedy as well as a circulatory stimulant. It first appears in a 14th-century Chinese herbal – the *Ben Cao Yan Yi Bu Yi*.

ACTIONS
antibacterial, hypotensive, peripheral vasodilator, cardiac tonic, lowers cholesterol levels

INDICATIONS
☻ to eliminate food stagnation and improve digestion
☻ to invigorate Blood circulation and clear Blood stagnation

USES
Shan Zha is used for digestive problems such as indigestion, abdominal bloating discomfort, and diarrhea, which are associated with food stagnation. It also helps to invigorate Blood and clear stasis, so is another of the remedies used for menstrual problems and heart disorders.

SHAN ZHU YU

PARTS USED
Fruit
TASTE
Sour
CHARACTER
Warm
MERIDIANS
Liver, Kidney

BOTANICAL NAME
Cornus officinalis
COMMON NAME
Dogwood, Japanese cornelian cherry

Shan Zhu Yu is another of the herbs listed by Shen Nong more than two thousand years ago. He regarded it as a wood in the "middle class," declaring that it "warms the center and expels cold and damp." Today, it is regarded primarily as an astringent herb to stop bleeding.

ACTIONS
antibacterial, antifungal, diuretic, hypotensive

INDICATIONS
☻ to replenish Liver and Kidney *Jing*
☻ to stop bleeding and excessive sweating

USES
Shan Zhu Yu is mainly used for urinary dysfunction associated with Kidney weakness, although as a *Jing* tonic is it is also included in remedies like *Liu Wei Di Huang Wan* (pills of six ingredients with rehmannia), which is used for scanty menstruation and, with minor changes, for menopausal problems.

CONTRAINDICATIONS
Avoid in excess syndromes.

CONTRAINDICATIONS
Use cautiously in cases of deficient Spleen and Stomach, and if there is acid regurgitation.

CONTRAINDICATIONS
Avoid with Fire symptoms and deficiency of Kidney yang. Do not combine it with *Jie Geng* or *Fang Feng*.

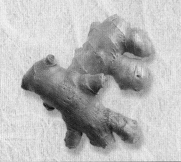

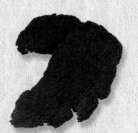

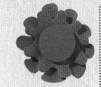

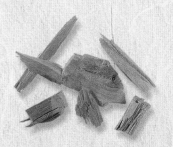

SHENG JIANG

PARTS USED
Root
TASTE
Pungent
CHARACTER
Warm
MERIDIANS
Lung, Spleen, Stomach

BOTANICAL NAME
Zingiber officinale
COMMON NAME
Fresh ginger

Sheng Jiang is fresh ginger and is mainly used as a warming remedy for Wind–Cold chills. This herb, when dried, becomes *Gan Jiang*, which has a more tonic action, helping to replenish yang and warm the Spleen and Stomach. The peel of fresh ginger root (*Sheng Jiang Pi*) is a diuretic.

ACTIONS
antiemetic, antispasmodic, antiseptic, carminative, circulatory stimulant, diaphoretic, expectorant, peripheral vasodilator. Topically, used as a rubefacient

INDICATIONS
◉ to release the exterior, strengthen *Wei Qi* and disperse Cold
◉ to warm the Middle *Jiao*
◉ to reduce the toxicity of other herbs

USES
Sheng Jiang is included mainly in remedies for chills, common colds, and coughs with thin watery phlegm. In the West, it is highly regarded as an anti-emetic, and in China it is also used to prevent vomiting – often in combination with *Ban Xia*.

SHU DI HUANG

PARTS USED
Tuberous root
TASTE
Sweet
CHARACTER
Slightly warm
MERIDIANS
Heart, Liver, Kidney

BOTANICAL NAME
Rehmannia glutinosa
COMMON NAME
Chinese foxglove

Shu Di Huang is a prepared form of the herb made by stir-frying the sliced tubers with wine. It is a major Blood tonic. The raw herb, *Sheng Di Huang*, is colder and it is sometimes cooked (without wine) to produce *Gan Di Huang*. Both of these forms are helpful for yin and Body Fluids, as well as being used to clear Heat.

ACTIONS
cardiotonic, diuretic, mild laxative, reduces blood sugar

INDICATIONS
◉ to nourish and tonify Blood
◉ to nourish Kidney yin and *Jing*

USES
Shu Di Huang is used in such blood disorders as anemia, irregular menstruation, and abnormal uterine bleeding. It is also an effective Kidney herb, helping to strengthen energies and combat the typical deficiency symptoms of low back pain and night sweats.

TAN XIANG

PARTS USED
Heartwood
TASTE
Pungent
CHARACTER
Warm
MERIDIANS
Spleen, Stomach, Lung, Heart

BOTANICAL NAME:
Santalum album
COMMON NAME
Sandalwood

Sandalwood is an important Ayurvedic herb that has been used in China since around 500 CE. In Europe, the oil is widely used in aromatherapy as a calming, relaxing remedy, but the heartwood is preferred in Chinese remedies.

ACTIONS
analgesic, antiseptic, antibacterial, antispasmodic, diuretic, sedative

INDICATIONS
◉ to move Stomach and Spleen *Qi* and improve digestion
◉ to dispel Cold
◉ to clear Blood stagnation and relieve pain

USES
Tan Xiang is used for abdominal bloating and spasms, as well as for indigestion – it is often combined with other carminative remedies like *Sha Ren*. It is also believed to clear Blood stasis, so is combined with herbs like *Dan Shen*, which is for treating angina pectoris and heart pains.

CONTRAINDICATIONS	CONTRAINDICATIONS	CONTRAINDICATIONS
Avoid in internal Heat syndromes.	Not to be used in cases of diarrhea or indigestion.	Avoid in cases of yin deficiency and excess Fire.

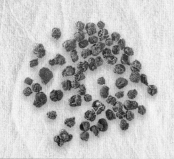
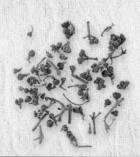
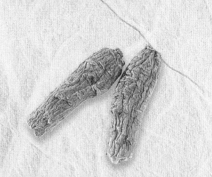

WU WEI ZI

PARTS USED
Fruit
TASTE
Sour
CHARACTER
Warm
MERIDIANS
Lung, Heart, Kidney

BOTANICAL NAME
Schisandra chinensis
COMMON NAME
Shisandra

A lthough the taste of *Wu Wei Zi* is generally given as "sour," the name means "five taste seeds" and it was once regarded as a combination of all five of the classic Chinese tastes.

ACTIONS
antibacterial, astringent, aphrodisiac, circulatory stimulant, digestive stimulant, expectorant, hypotensive, sedative, tonic, uterine stimulant

INDICATIONS
☻ to replenish *Qi*, especially Lung *Qi*
☻ to promote Body Fluids
☻ to tonify Kidney and Heart; to calm the spirit (*Shen*)
☻ to stop excessive sweating

USES
Wu Wei Zi has an impressive array of uses – for coughs, skin rashes, chronic diarrhea, insomnia, and severe shock. It is used with *Gan Jiang* for coughs and wheezing, with *Bu Gu Zhi* in Kidney deficiency, and with *Huang Qi* for deficient yang. Its five tastes reputedly help all five *Zang* organs, and it can also be used for skin irritation.

WU ZHU YU

PARTS USED
Fruits
TASTE
Pungent, bitter
CHARACTER
Hot, slightly toxic
MERIDIANS
Spleen, Stomach, Liver, Kidney

BOTANICAL NAME
Evodia rutacarpa
COMMON NAME
Evodia

W u Zhu Yu is a toxic herb that has been used as a warming remedy for cold conditions since the days of Shen Nong. He describes it as "warming the center" and dispelling Wind. The plant is traditionally mixed with licorice water to reduce its toxicity.

ACTIONS
antibacterial, antiparasitic, analgesic, raises body temperature, respiratory stimulant, uterine stimulant

INDICATIONS
☻ to warm the Spleen and Stomach
☻ to dispel Cold and relieve pain
☻ to reverse the flow of *Qi*

USES
Wu Zhu Yu is used for pain and vomiting associated with internal Cold or Phlegm, as well as for the upward movement of rebellious *Qi,* which can cause vomiting and acid regurgitation. It is combined with fresh ginger (*Sheng Jiang*) for stomach pain and vomiting, and with dried ginger (*Gan Jiang*) for Cold Stomach syndromes.

XI YANG SHEN

PARTS USED
Root
TASTE
Sweet, slightly bitter
CHARACTER
Cool
MERIDIANS
Heart, Lung, Kidney

BOTANICAL NAME:
Panax quinquifolius
COMMON NAME
American ginseng

A merican ginseng was "discovered" by Jesuit priests in Canada in the early 18th century and, by 1765, it had been logged by Chinese herbalists in the **Ben Cao Gang Mu Shi Yi** ("**Omissions from the Grand Materia Medica**") by Zhao Xue Min . The plant rapidly became a valuable export – collected by backwoodsmen like Daniel Boone and shipped to China in huge quantities during the 19th century.

ACTIONS
hormonal action, sedative

INDICATIONS
☻ to nourish *Qi*, Body Fluids, and yin
☻ to nurture Lung yin

USES
American ginseng is very similar to its Korean cousin, although it is rather more supportive for yin and Body Fluids. It is used in China for chronic coughs associated with Lung deficiency, and with low-grade fevers. It is also used for fatigue and debility in chronic disorders.

CONTRAINDICATIONS
Avoid in cases of internal Heat and superficial syndromes.

CONTRAINDICATIONS
Avoid in cases of yin deficiency and excess Fire.

CONTRAINDICATIONS
Avoid where there are symptoms of Cold and Damp in the Stomach.

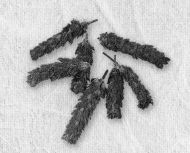

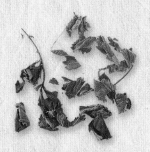

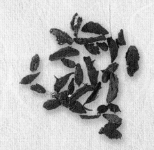

XIA KU CAO

PARTS USED
Flower spike
TASTE
Bitter, pungent
CHARACTER
Cool
MERIDIANS
Lung, Gall Bladder

BOTANICAL NAME
Prunella vulgaris
COMMON NAME
Self-heal

XIAN HE CAO

PARTS USED
Aerial parts
TASTE
Bitter, astringent
CHARACTER
Neutral
MERIDIANS
Lung, Spleen, Liver

BOTANICAL NAME
Agrimonia pilosa
COMMON NAME
Agrimony

XIANG FU

PARTS USED
Tuber
TASTE
Pungent, slightly bitter
CHARACTER
Neutral
MERIDIANS
Liver, Stomach

BOTANICAL NAME
Cyperus rotundus
COMMON NAME
Nutgrass

Self-heal is a common European wildflower, traditionally used in folk medicine as a wound herb – hence its English name. The Chinese see it as an important cooling remedy for the Liver and it can be very effective for calming hyperactive children (who are often suffering from Liver Fire syndromes).

ACTIONS
antibacterial, hypotensive, diuretic, astringent, wound herb

INDICATIONS
◉ to clear Heat from the Liver
◉ to dissipate nodules

USES
Liver Heat is associated with problems like eye inflammations, headaches, vertigo, and irritability, and *Xia Ku Cao* can be effective for all these sorts of symptoms – often combined with *Ju Hua* or *Xiang Fu*. It is also used for clearing swellings in mastitis, mumps, goiter, and lymphatic disorders, which are associated with constrained Liver *Qi*.

European agrimony is a common wound herb and remedy for diarrhea. Its close Chinese remedy is also used as a styptic to stop bleeding, as well as having notable antibacterial properties for treating a wide range of infectious conditions.

ACTIONS
antibacterial, antiparasitic, anti-inflammatory, analgesic, astringent, hemostatic, hypertensive

INDICATIONS
◉ to stop bleeding
◉ to expel parasites
◉ to combat Fire Poisons as a detoxicant

USES
Xian He Cao is used for problems like nosebleeds, spitting, coughing, or vomiting blood, blood in the urine, abnormal uterine bleeding, and any sort of hemorrhage – much as is its European counterpart. It is also used in suppositories for intestinal parasites, and taken for boils, carbuncles, malaria, dysentery, and vaginal infections.

Xiang Fu literally means "aromatic attachment," which describes this highly scented plant. This herb is classified as a *Qi* regulator, and can be prepared with vinegar, to enhance its pain-killing effect, or salt, to help it moisten Blood and Body Fluids.

ACTIONS
analgesic, antibacterial, antispasmodic for the uterus

INDICATIONS
◉ to promote the circulation of *Qi* and smooth Liver *Qi*
◉ to relieve menstrual pains

USES
Xiang Fu is used for various digestive problems and menstrual disorders, including both colicky and period pains, abdominal bloating, indigestion, and abnormal uterine bleeding. It is the main herb in *Xiang Fu San* (which also contains *Zi Su Ye, Chen Pi,* and *Gan Cao*), and is a warming remedy for both Wind–Cold and internal *Qi* stagnation.

CONTRAINDICATIONS
Avoid if the Spleen or Stomach are weak.

CONTRAINDICATIONS
Avoid in Heat and Fire conditions.

CONTRAINDICATIONS
Avoid in Heat syndromes associated with yin deficiency.

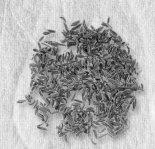

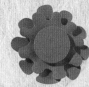

XIAO HUI XIANG

PARTS USED
Seeds
TASTE
Pungent
CHARACTER
Warm

BOTANICAL NAME
Foeniculum vulgare
COMMON NAM
Fennel

MERIDIANS
Stomach, Liver, Kidney

F ennel seeds have been used in China since the 11th century. As in the West, they are considered an important warming remedy for stomach problems, but they are also believed to affect the Liver and encourage energy flows.

ACTIONS
anti-inflammatory, carminative, circulatory stimulant, galactogogue, mild expectorant, diuretic

INDICATIONS
☙ to regulate *Qi* and alleviate pain
☙ to warm the Stomach and Middle *Jiao*

USES
Xiao Hui Xiang is often combined with *Rou Gui, Sheng Jiang,* or *Hou Po* for problems associated with Cold in the Stomach. Typical symptoms include colicky pains, poor appetite, indigestion, and vomiting.

XIN YI HUA

PARTS USED
Flower, flower bud
TASTE
Pungent
CHARACTER
Warm

BOTANICAL NAME
Magnolia liliflora
COMMON NAME
Lily-flowered magnolia

MERIDIAN
Lung, Stomach

X in Yi Hua – another of the West's ornamental trees – is listed by Shen Nong as a "superior wood" that is useful, among other things, for "pain in the brain and black patches on the face." The herb is mainly used for exterior conditions, notably Wind and Cold, although Shen Nong also used it for certain Heat problems.

ACTIONS
analgesic, anticatarrhal, antifungal, hypotensive, sedative, uterine stimulant

INDICATIONS
☙ to expel Wind and Cold
☙ to open the nasal passages

USES
Xin Yin Hua is often combined with *Cang Er Zi* for nasal congestion and sinus headaches, while adding *Ju Hua* helps sinusitis. Mixtures containing *Bo He* and *Huang Qin* are preferred for Heat conditions. *Xin Yi San* is a powder used for a blocked nose with severe catarrh; it also includes *Gao Ben, Fang Feng,* and *Chuang Xiong.*

XING REN

PARTS USED
Seeds
TASTE
Bitter
CHARACTER
Slightly warm, slightly toxic

BOTANICAL NAME
Prunus armeniaca
COMMON NAME
Bitter apricot

MERIDIANS
Lung, Large Intestine

X ing Ren, used as a medicinal herb since the 6th century, is an important remedy to relieve coughs and wheezing. Modern research has confirmed that it is efficacious, although, as apricot seeds contain hydrocyanic acid, high doses can be toxic; fatalities have been reported from adults eating sixty pieces and children only ten.

ACTIONS
antitussive, anti-asthmatic, antibacterial, antiparasitic, analgesic

INDICATIONS
☙ to relieve coughs and stop wheezing
☙ to lubricate the Intestines

USES
Xing Ren is suitable for many sorts of coughs. It is combined with *Zi Su Ye* for dry coughs associated with Wind–Cold and with *Sang Ye* for nonproductive coughs caused by Wind–Heat. With *Ma Huang* it is used for wheezy conditions; with *Huo Ma Ren* it makes an effective laxative for deficient, dry Intestines.

CONTRAINDICATIONS
Use cautiously in deficient yin syndromes.

CONTRAINDICATIONS
Avoid in excess Fire conditions associated with yin deficiency.

CONTRAINDICATIONS
Avoid in cases of coughs caused by deficient yin.

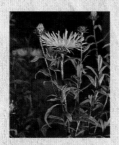
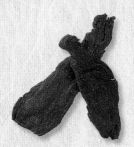
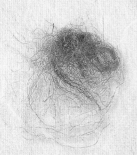

XUAN FU HUA

PARTS USED
Flowerheads
TASTE
Salty
CHARACTER
Warm
MERIDIANS
Lung, Spleen, Stomach, Large Intestine

BOTANICAL NAME
Inula brittanica
COMMON NAME
Japanese elecampane

While the root of European elecampane (*I. helenium*) is preferred as an effective expectorant and tonic, the Chinese use the flowers of a related species instead. Shen Nong recommended it for Damp and Cold problems, giving it an alternative name of *Sheng Zhan*, which means "profound clearness."

ACTIONS
antibacterial, nervous stimulant, digestive stimulant

INDICATIONS
◉ to redirect upwardly flowing Lung and Stomach *Qi*
◉ to resolve stagnation of Phlegm in the Lung

USES
Xuan Fu Hua is preferred for coughs with copious, thick sputum, as well as disordered Stomach *Qi* problems, which may involve vomiting and hiccups. It is combined with *Ren Shen*, *Ban Xia*, *Shen Jiang*, and *Da Zao* for Stomach *Qi* problems.

XUAN SHEN

PARTS USED
Root
TASTE
Bitter, salty
CHARACTER
Cold
MERIDIANS
Lung, Stomach, Kidney

BOTANICAL NAME
Scrophularia ningpoensis
COMMON NAME
Ningpo figwort

Xuan Shen was also included in Shen Nong's herbal and is an extremely effective herb for clearing the Fire Poisons. Shen Nong suggests that it can strengthen Kidney *Qi* and brighten the eyes. He also recommended it for problems like mastitis during breast-feeding.

ACTIONS
antibacterial, antiviral, cardiotonic, hypotensive, hypoglycemic.

INDICATIONS
◉ to nourish yin and *Jing*
◉ to clear the Heat and Fire Poisons
◉ to soften and dissipate hard swellings and nodules

USES
Xuan Shen is good for all sorts of deep-seated abscesses (including dental abscesses), acute swellings in the throat, and irritant rashes associated with infections when it is combined with *Mu Dan Pi*. It can help dry coughs and, as a yin tonic, is also good for insomnia and palpitations following feverish disorders.

YU MI XU

PARTS USE
Styles and stigmata
TASTE
Sweet
CHARACTER
Neutral
MERIDIAN
Liver, Gall Bladder, Urinary Bladder, Small Intestine

BOTANICAL NAME
Zea mays
COMMON NAME
Cornsilk

As in Western herbal medicine, the Chinese use cornsilk mainly as a soothing diuretic. The name means "jade rice whiskers," and the herb was first mentioned in a Sichuan herbal of unknown date, suggesting that this American plant was introduced via Southern China.

ACTIONS
diuretic, demulcent, antilithic, mild stimulant

INDICATIONS
◉ to promote urination
◉ to benefit the Gall Bladder and clear jaundice

USES
Yu Mi Xu is a soothing diuretic for a range of urinary problems. It helps to clear both urinary stones and gallstones, and will also help to stop bleeding. In Chinese folk tradition, it is used in mouthwashes for bleeding gums and also to lower blood sugar levels in cases of diabetes.

CONTRAINDICATIONS
Avoid excessive use in deficiency syndromes.

CONTRAINDICATIONS
Avoid in cases of diarrhea.

CONTRAINDICATIONS
None noted.

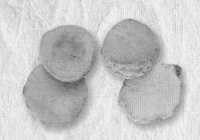

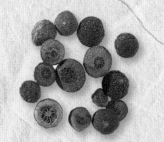

ZE XIE

PARTS USED
Tuber
TASTE
Sweet
CHARACTER
Cold
MERIDIANS
Kidney, Urinary Bladder

BOTANICAL NAME
Alisma plantago-aquatica
COMMON NAME
Water plantain

Shen Nong included *Ze Xie* in his "superior class of herbs," declaring that it would "boost the *Qi* … and make one fat and strong," as well as prolong life and "enable one to walk over water." Rather more moderate claims are more normal today. The herb is an effective diuretic and Liver remedy.

ACTIONS
antibacterial, diuretic, hypotensive, lowers blood sugar and cholesterol

INDICATIONS
☺ to regulate Water metabolism and resolve Dampness
☺ to eliminate Heat and Dampness in the Lower *Jiao*

USES
Ze Xie is used for edema and urinary dysfunction associated with poor Water metabolism and Damp. It is also now known to reduce fatty deposits in the Liver, and is used in remedies like *Liu Wei Di Huang Wan* (*see* pages 48–49).

CONTRAINDICATIONS
Avoid in deficient Kidney yang.

ZHE BEI MU

PARTS USED
Bulb
TASTE
Bitter
CHARACTER
Cold
MERIDIANS
Lung, Heart

BOTANICAL NAME
Fritillaria verticillata
COMMON NAME
Fritillary

Zhe Bei Mu is one of the more important herbs to clear Hot Phlegm, which is responsible for acute Lung problems and productive coughs with thick, yellow sputum. Several varieties of fritillary are used in Chinese medicine – e.g., *Chuan Bei Mu* (*F. cirrhosa*) is most suitable for nonproductive coughs.

ACTIONS
antitussive, hypotensive, muscle relaxant

INDICATIONS
☺ to clear and transform Heat and Phlegm
☺ to resolve coughs
☺ to disperse hard lumps and swellings

USES
Zhe Bei Mu is used for respiratory problems, such as acute bronchitis. It is often combined with *Lian Qiao* and *Niu Bang Zi*. For abscesses and swelling, it is more likely to be used with *Xuan Shen* or *Xia Ku Cao*.

CONTRAINDICATIONS
Avoid in conditions with deficient Spleen patterns.

ZHI SHI

PARTS USED
Immature fruit
TASTE
Sour, bitter
CHARACTER
Slightly cold
MERIDIANS
Spleen, Stomach

BOTANICAL NAME
Citrus aurantium
COMMON NAME
Bitter orange

Zhi Shi is the unripe fruit of bitter orange, while *Zhi Ke* is the ripe fruit. Both are used in very similar ways, although the ripe fruit is rather milder in action. The fruits have been used as carminatives and digestive remedies since the days of Shen Nong.

ACTIONS
antihistamine, carminative, diuretic, hypertensive

INDICATIONS
☺ to disperse stagnant *Qi*
☺ to direct the *Qi* downward and move stool
☺ to resolve hard swellings

USES
Zhi Shi is commonly used. It is included in remedies with herbs like *Hou Po* and *Da Huang* for food stagnation – typified by indigestion, constipation, or abdominal swellings. It is also used with *Bai Shao* for pain due to *Qi* or Blood obstruction.

CONTRAINDICATIONS
Use cautiously in pregnancy, where *Qi* is weak, or with Cold Deficient Stomach problems.

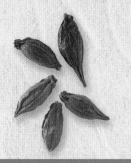
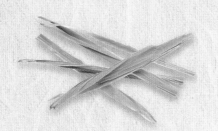
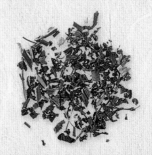

ZHI ZI

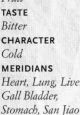

PARTS USED
Fruit
TASTE
Bitter
CHARACTER
Cold
MERIDIANS
Heart, Lung, Liver, Gall Bladder, Stomach, San Jiao

BOTANICAL NAME
Gardenia jasminoides
COMMON NAME
Gardenia

Zhi Zi has been used to clear Hot conditions since the days of Shen Nong. The herb is used raw for Heat and Dampness, and can be stir-fried for Heat in the Blood, or carbonized to improve its styptic action.

ACTIONS
antibacterial, antifungal, antiparasitic, cholagogue, hypotensive, laxative, sedative

INDICATIONS
◉ to clear Heat and relieve irritability
◉ to drain Damp Heat
◉ to clear Heat and Fire poisons from the Blood

USES
Gardenia fruits are an important remedy for quelling Fire, and they are used for high fevers, inflamed eyes, or acute hepatitis. They are used with *Mu Dan Pi* for Heat caused by deficient Liver Blood, which may include period pains with headaches, and with *Shen Di Huang* for Heat-induced hemorrhaging.

ZHU RU

PARTS USED
Stem shavings
TASTE
Sweet
CHARACTER
Slightly cold
MERIDIANS
Lung, Stomach, Gall Bladder

BOTANICAL NAME
Phylostachys nigra
COMMON NAME:
Bamboo

Various parts of the bamboo plant are used medicinally. As well as the shavings (taken from the stem with the outer green skin removed), there is *Zhu Li*, which is the dried sap, and *Zhu Ye*, the leaves. All are sweet and cold, and are mainly used to clear Phlegm and Heat, and to encourage Body Fluid production.

ACTIONS
antibacterial

INDICATIONS
◉ to clear Phlegm and Heat in the Lungs
◉ to clear Heat from the Stomach and stop vomiting
◉ to cool the Blood and stop bleeding

USES
Zhi Ru is used with *Dang Shen* and *Gan Cao* for cases of deficient Stomach *Qi*, and with *Ban Xia*, *Chen Pi*, *Zhi Shi*, *Fu Ling*, *Gan Cao*, and *Da Zao* in *Wen Dan Tang* (gall bladder warming decoction) for disharmonies between Liver and Stomach leading to insomnia and vomiting.

ZI SU YE

PARTS USED
Leaf
TASTE
Pungent
CHARACTER
Warm
MERIDIANS
Lung, Spleen

BOTANICAL NAME
Perilla frutescens
COMMON NAME
Purple perilla

Perilla is a popular Eastern culinary herb that is occasionally found in Asian supermarkets in Europe. It is warming and combats the cold nature of certain foods. The leaves (*Zi Su Ye*) and fruits (*Zi Su Zi*) are used for Lung and digestive disorders. The stems (*Su Geng*) are used to redirect *Qi*.

ACTIONS
antibacterial, antitussive, diaphoretic, expectorant

INDICATIONS
◉ to redirect *Qi* downward and relieve coughing
◉ to combat external Wind and Cold
◉ to promote the flow of *Qi* in the Spleen/Stomach
◉ to lubricate the Intestines

USES
Zhi Su Ye is used with *Zhe Bei Mu* and *Ban Xia* for coughs and wheezing, or with *Huo Ma Ren* for constipation associated with dryness. For Wind–Cold conditions it is often combined with *Chen Pi*, *Xiang Fu*, and *Gan Cao* in *Xiang Su San*.

CONTRAINDICATIONS
Avoid in cases of diarrhea.

CONTRAINDICATIONS
Avoid in cases of coughs caused by Cold, and diarrhea due to Spleen deficiency.

CONTRAINDICATIONS
Avoid in feverish diseases and where there is *Qi* deficiency.

UNUSUAL INGREDIENTS

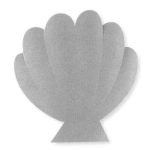

*C*hina's use of body parts from animals of endangered species quite rightly shocks the Western world. Bear gallbladders, tiger bones, geckos, seahorses, and water buffalo gallstones are part of this less attractive face of Chinese medicine.

ALTERNATIVES TO PLANTS

The range of traditional Chinese "drugs" has always gone far beyond the plant kingdom. Shen Nong provides a long list of minerals and precious stones, as well as a gruesome collection of animal parts, which have a clearly defined therapeutic action.

Some are relatively acceptable:
• *Xue Yu Tan* – charred human hair – is used today as a diuretic and to stop bleeding. Shen Nong also suggested it as a remedy for epilepsy in children.

• *Ji Nei Jin* – the lining of chicken gizzards – is used for food stagnation problems and to contain *Jing* in cases of bedwetting and frequent urination.
• *Hai Ge Ke* – clam shells – are used to clear Heat and redirect *Qi* down.
• *Wu Zei Gu* – cuttlefish bones – are used as an astringent to stop bleeding and to support the Kidneys and *Jing*.
• *Dong Chong Xia Cao* – a fungus which grows on the nose of a moth caterpillar, and the larva – are used as a yang tonic for the Lungs and

Kidneys. Fortunately, Western herbal suppliers have developed ways of breeding the fungus on cereal substrates, so afflicted caterpillars are no longer required. The caterpillars were traditionally cooked with duck, chicken, pork, or fish to make a tonic stew to strengthen the *Wei Qi*.

BELOW **The range of traditional Chinese "drugs" has always reached far beyond what the plant kingdom can offer.**

RIGHT **Animal parts used in Chinese medicine may strike Westerners as the unpalatable side of traditional treatment.**

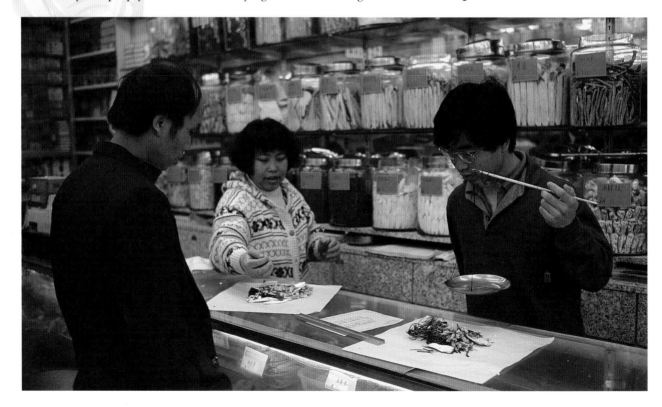

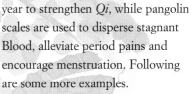

LESS PALATABLE OPTIONS

Other remedies may strike Westerners as less savory, either because the remedy seems revolting or the slaughter or "farming" of wild animals to provide the necessary body parts is unacceptable. In all cases, Western therapists would argue that there are perfectly adequate plant or mineral alternatives to these animal remedies – although the Chinese tend to disagree.

A visit to any Chinese food market will reveal an assortment of puppies, cats, tortoises, frogs, and even pangolins, intended not as family pets but for the next meal. Dog meat, for example, is supposed to help yang, and is eaten at particular times of the year to strengthen *Qi*, while pangolin scales are used to disperse stagnant Blood, alleviate period pains and encourage menstruation. Following are some more examples.

• *Ye Ming Sha* – bat feces – are used as a Liver tonic and eye remedy, and cooked with various animal livers in a traditional stew for night blindness.

• *Niu Huang* – water buffalo gallstones – are listed by Shen Nong as a remedy for Phlegm and Liver Wind, and are still used in this way.

• *Hai Ma* – seahorses – are used to tonify the Kidneys, especially in elderly people suffering from debility.

• *Ge Jie* – gecko – is used to tonify Kidney yang and the Lungs.

• *Can Sha* – silkworm feces – are used to expel Wind–Damp.

• *Hu Gu* – tiger bones – are used to disperse Wind–Cold and Wind–Dampness in painful joint conditions.

• *Hai Gou She* – seal testes – are used to strengthen yang and *Jing,* and are often combined with *Dong Chong Xia Cao* as a remedy for impotence.

• *Xiong Dan* – bear's gall bladder – is used to clear Heat and Fire poisons, calm Liver Fire, and reduce pain and swelling in sprains and fractures.

• *She Xiang* – navel gland secretions from the musk deer – is used as a strongly aromatic substance to revive the senses in convulsions and coma, and to stimulate the birth of stillborns and expulsion of the placenta.

• *Lu Rong* – the velvet of young deer antlers – is used to tonify the Kidneys and *Du Mai* (*see* page 30).

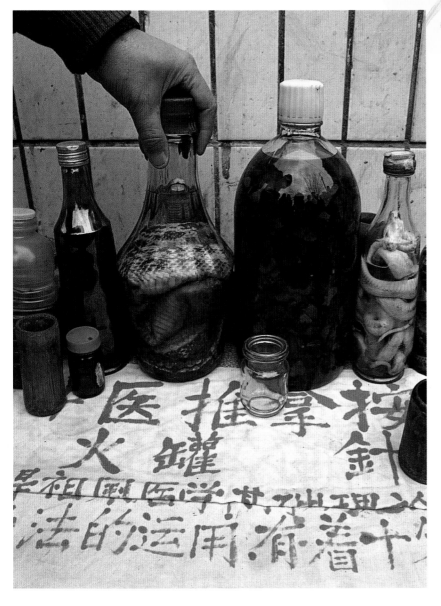

THE ORIGINS OF ACUPUNCTURE

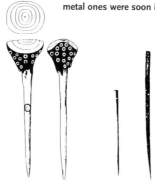

*A*cupuncture is believed to have originated at least four thousand years ago from early methods of lancing boils and drawing fluid from swollen joints. In Paleolithic times, stone needles were used, to be replaced by bone and bamboo during the Neolithic period.

FROM FLINT TO STAINLESS STEEL

Just as Shen Nong is credited with the discovery of herbal medicine, so the *Nei Jing Su Wen* of Huang Di, the Yellow Emperor, is the first-known text to describe acupuncture.

In those times, the needles used were made of flint. The Chinese character for sharp flint needles, *Bian*, is believed to be the origin of the modern Chinese term *Bi*, which means a painful disease. For example, "*Bi* syndrome" is how Chinese medicine defines the different forms of arthritis.

However, acupuncture is much more than simply treating pain. It concerns rebalancing energy flows and moving stagnating *Qi* – or, as the Yellow Emperor put it, "acupuncture is applied in order to supply what is lacking and in order to drain off excessive fullness."

Originally, acupuncture was largely to do with lancing boils and relieving sites of infection, flint needles being applied as and where needed, with practitioners having little idea of meridians or acu points. Over the centuries, these flint needles were replaced by metal needles. Nine different shapes are described in the *Nei Jing*, ranging from an arrowhead

for superficial pricking to a large, long needle for puncturing joints. Given acupuncture's origins, it is not surprising that a key member of the set was a sword-like needle for draining abscesses. Gold and silver were generally preferred, with yellow gold regarded as more yang in character than gray silver needles. Today, most modern acupuncturists use stainless steel needles ranging from around 13 mm (0.5 in) in length to 130 mm (5 in), and from 0.25 mm to about 0.5 mm in diameter. The thicker needles are generally used for fleshy areas, such as the soles of the feet, and the finer ones for thin skin as on the face or arms.

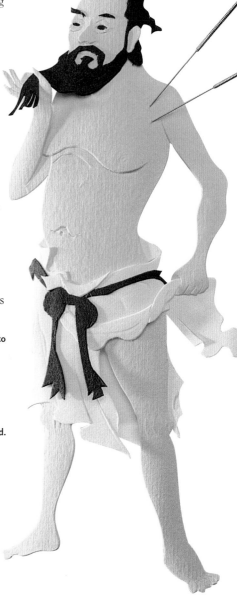

RIGHT **Acupuncture dates back to the days of the Yellow Emperor, with many surviving early texts describing the technique.**

BELOW **The first needles were made from splinters of flint, but metal ones were soon introduced.**

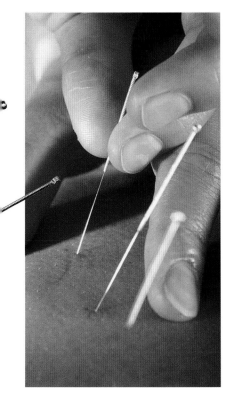

LEFT **Various techniques have developed over the centuries, including twisting or stirring the needles.**

the major points used today. By the sixth century, when China's first medical school – the Imperial Medical College – was founded, acupuncture was an established and highly formalized therapy.

Over the following centuries, more points were identified, and meridians codified, as acupuncture became a familiar and widely used tool throughout China. With the arrival of European medicine and missionaries, however, it gradually fell from favor – coming to be regarded by the Emperors as a "bar to progress." In 1822, it was dropped from the Imperial College curriculum and by 1929 had been completely banned. It was only during the 1950s, with the revival of interest in traditional Chinese therapies then being encouraged by the communist government, that acupuncture clinics began to open once more. They stimulated interest, not only in the old treatments, but also in a new scientific approach to acupuncture therapy.

DEFINING THE MERIDIANS

By the time the *Nei Jing* came to be formally written down (some time between 1000 and 220 BCE – long after the Yellow Emperor, who lived around 2697–2579 BCE), the main meridians had been defined, and acupuncture points – or spots – identified. These were not the only points likely to be treated, however, and the *Nei Jing* advises practitioners to "puncture the tender spot" – much as modern practitioners, who still try to ease pain by pressing on painful areas.

The **Nei Jing** and the rather later **Zhenjiu Jiayijing** ("**Classic of Acupuncture and Moxabustion**") written by Huangfu Mi (214–282 CE) list 349 acupuncture points – most of

NAMING THE POINTS

The 361 main acu points are described in terms of their location on specific meridians that are numbered from the start of the channel. Standard shorthand uses an abbreviation for the therapeutic location and point number, although each point also has its own name. The first Lung meridian point, LU1, for example, is known as *Zhongfu*.

Name of meridian	Abbreviation	No. of acu points
Lung	LU	11
Large intestine	LI	20
Spleen	SP	21
Stomach	ST	45
Heart	HT	9
Small Intestine	SI	19
Urinary Bladder	UB	67
Kidney	KD	27
Liver	LV	14
Gall Bladder	GB	44
Pericardium	PC	9
San Jiao/Triple Burner	SJ	23
Governing Vessel (*Du Mai*)	GV	28
Conception Vessel (*Ren Mai*)	CV	24

USING ACUPUNCTURE TODAY

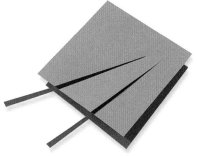

*A*lthough, to many Westerners, acupuncture seems the archetypal Eastern therapy, in China it is far less popular than herbs. Typically, patients given herbal prescriptions will outnumber those recommended acupuncture by about eight to one.

MANIPULATING *QI*

Acupuncture treatment is concerned with manipulating the *Qi* flow through the meridians in order to simulate movement and clear stagnation. It can be helpful where there is an imbalance in the *Zang Fu* organs in helping to restore harmony.

For superficial syndromes affecting the exterior, acupuncture may produce rapid relief, but for interior problems, a longer treatment is usually needed. In China it is not unusual for people with serious ailments to receive up to 2000 treatment sessions.

Treatments are often given on a daily basis in courses of 12 or more. Western patients are unlikely to visit their therapists so regularly.

In China, acupuncture is seen as additional to herbal medicine, and treatment is likely to be prescribed when pain is being experienced. In the West, practitioners tend to train as acupuncturists rather than Traditional Chinese Medicine doctors. Many recommend herbal medicines, but the approach may be formulaic – using prepared herbs, rather than adapting the prescription to suit the individual.

WHERE ACUPUNCTURE CAN HELP

Although acupuncture is used for a wide and growing range of ailments in the West, it is worth remembering that traditionally it was not the first choice for many problems. It main use is in stimulating, balancing, and moving *Qi,* and if these sorts of deficiencies are not an aspect of someone's problem, it may be inappropriate.

Acupuncture can be helpful for sprains and other muscular/joint injuries, and it can provide relief from osteoarthritis for six months or more,

RIGHT **Various of the 361 acu points are treated for a wide range of conditions.**

UB13 Feishu *is located on the 3rd thoracic vertebra. It may be treated for lung problems such as pneumonia.*

UB18 Ganshu *is located on the 9th thoracic vertebra. It may be treated for liver problems such as hepatitis.*

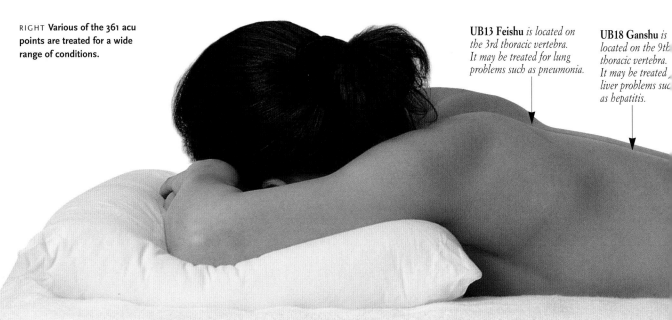

although treatment does need to be repeated at intervals. It is generally not suitable for rheumatoid arthritis during the inflammatory stage but can be useful for pain relief when osteoarthritis then develops in the damaged joint.

Many acupuncturists report that up to 95% of headaches can be successfully treated. Acupuncture is also successful for migraine, and often gives very long-term relief, leaving sufferers migraine-free for years.

Nerve pains (neuralgia) also respond well, and acupuncture can be successful in treating the sort of nerve pains that can develop following shingles (*Herpes zoster*).

There tends to be a more mixed reaction to acupuncture used for digestive and respiratory problems, although success rates of 50% or more have been reported for conditions such as bronchitis and inflammatory bowel disorders. Often, however, there are more suitable therapies with a greater chance of success for curing problems.

Studies also suggest that acupuncture can be effective in cases of angina pectoris (cure rates of up to 80% have been claimed), although, as with other chronic conditions, the treatment course needs to be repeated two or three times a year.

Medical reports from China also suggest significant success with stroke victims and in cases of paralysis. In many, acupuncture is likely to be only one aspect of treatment, which probably also will include *Qigong*, massage, and herbal remedies.

Acupuncture is also extremely helpful after surgery and helps to re-establish *Qi* flows in the affected meridians.

NEEDLING TECHNIQUES

Methods used in acupuncture treatment vary. Much depends on the individual patient. Needles will be inserted more deeply and vigorously in fleshy people than in thin, wiry ones, for example.

Needles are generally inserted lightly into the skin and its immediate underlying layer of fat or flesh. However, they may be pushed deeper into fleshy areas like the buttock.

The needles are usually left in for about twenty minutes, but they could stay in for an hour or more. Some ear acupuncturists will also leave a small ear seed in place between treatments to maintain pressure on the point.

Practitioners may move needles occasionally to stimulate acu points. Vigorous movement stirs stagnant *Qi*, for example, and a twisting or flicking motion strengthens the *Qi* flow.

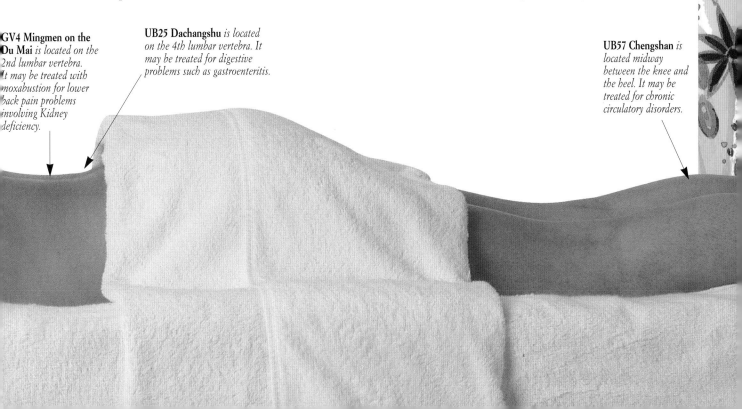

GV4 Mingmen on the Du Mai *is located on the 2nd lumbar vertebra. It may be treated with moxabustion for lower back pain problems involving Kidney deficiency.*

UB25 Dachangshu *is located on the 4th lumbar vertebra. It may be treated for digestive problems such as gastroenteritis.*

UB57 Chengshan *is located midway between the knee and the heel. It may be treated for chronic circulatory disorders.*

EAR ACUPUNCTURE AND MOXABUSTION

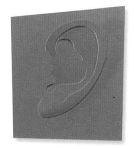

*A*lthough the Nei Jing *records that "the ear is the place where all the channels meet," ear acupuncture is one of the newer forms of the therapy that have developed in the past fifty years.*

A NEW APPROACH

The system of using the ear as a mirror of the body's organs for acupuncture treatment was largely formalized in France in the 1950s by Dr. Paul Nogier. Since 1959, it has also been used in China, largely for pain relief.

Some 54 points, mostly on the front of the ear, have been identified. These each correspond to one of the body's organs. Some of them reflect a modern view of anatomy, as with acu point 27, which signifies the sciatic nerve, while others reflect traditional Chinese concepts, such as number 25, the *Shenmen* or spirit gate, usually ascribed to HT7 and used for treating heart disease.

Ear acupuncture is popular in the West and has become a fashionable therapy for those attempting to give up smoking, with reports suggesting that about 40% of smokers can give up their habit completely within six months of using the technique.

It is contraindicated in pregnancy and can be inappropriate for the elderly or debilitated.

Ear acupuncture should be used with caution by those suffering from high blood pressure.

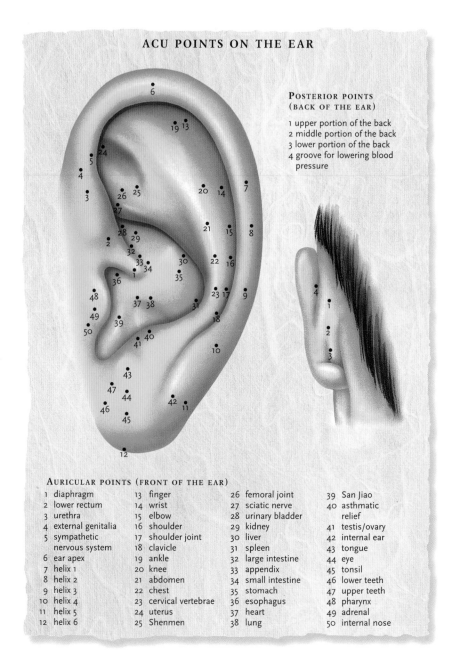

ACU POINTS ON THE EAR

POSTERIOR POINTS (BACK OF THE EAR)

1 upper portion of the back
2 middle portion of the back
3 lower portion of the back
4 groove for lowering blood pressure

AURICULAR POINTS (FRONT OF THE EAR)

1 diaphragm	13 finger	26 femoral joint	39 San Jiao
2 lower rectum	14 wrist	27 sciatic nerve	40 asthmatic relief
3 urethra	15 elbow	28 urinary bladder	
4 external genitalia	16 shoulder	29 kidney	41 testis/ovary
5 sympathetic nervous system	17 shoulder joint	30 liver	42 internal ear
	18 clavicle	31 spleen	43 tongue
6 ear apex	19 ankle	32 large intestine	44 eye
7 helix 1	20 knee	33 appendix	45 tonsil
8 helix 2	21 abdomen	34 small intestine	46 lower teeth
9 helix 3	22 chest	35 stomach	47 upper teeth
10 helix 4	23 cervical vertebrae	36 esophagus	48 pharynx
11 helix 5	24 uterus	37 heart	49 adrenal
12 helix 6	25 Shenmen	38 lung	50 internal nose

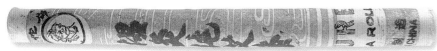

Moxa stick

MOXABUSTION

While most acupuncture simply involves inserting needles into the skin at the various acupuncture points, moxabustion is designed to apply heat to these same points using burning *moxa* (dried leaf of mugwort, *Artemisia vulgaris*).

The *moxa* is supplied either in tiny cones, sticks – large cigar-like tubes made from the herb – or as a "wool" that can be twisted onto the end of an acupuncture needle, which is then inserted as normal and lit. Loose *moxa* is also sometimes burned in a box placed on the body to help spread the heat over a larger area.

Moxabustion may be "direct" where it is burned on the body in cones or acupuncture needles, or "indirect" where the *moxa* is burned above the skin – by holding a stick 2.5 cm (1 in) over the area – or where some other substance, such as ginger or salt, is placed between the skin and the burning *moxa*.

Moxabustion is used for diseases associated with cold and damp – such as certain forms of arthritis and back pains. Moxabustion is never used if the patient has a fever or is suffering from a "hot" condition. Direct moxabustion with the herb left burning on the skin can cause scars and is never used for the face or head, or applied close to important organs, arteries or bones. In pregnancy, moxabustion treatment is never applied to the lower abdomen.

BELOW **Direct moxabustion treatment involves the burning of *moxa* on acupuncture needles.**

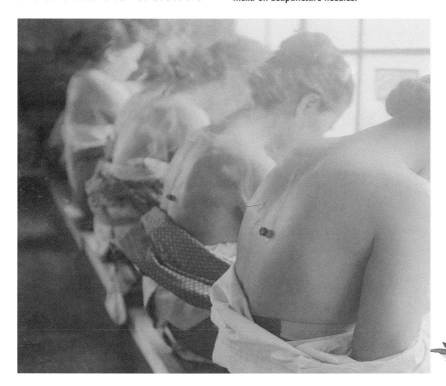

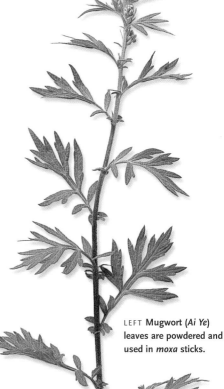

LEFT **Mugwort (*Ai Ye*) leaves are powdered and used in *moxa* sticks.**

OTHER TRADITIONAL CHINESE THERAPIES

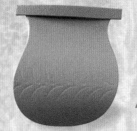

lthough acupuncture and Chinese herbal remedies are better known in the West, many other therapies have also evolved over the years. These, too, go back to the Yellow Emperor and early Chinese influences.

REGIONAL DIFFERENCES

It is believed that the diversity of traditional Chinese therapies owes much to the distinctive regional differences of early Chinese medicine and are as much a matter of geography as anything else. China was, and is, a vast country, and four thousand years ago travel was slow and limited. The Yellow Emperor, in his *Nei Jing Su Wen*, was the first to describe these regional differences.

He argues that in the hot, humid east of China, "ulcers" are the most common affliction and must be treated with acupuncture using flint needles. Some commentators assert that this suggests acupuncture originated from the need to lance the abscesses that would have been commonplace in such climates.

In the mountainous, wind-swept regions of the west of the country, there were fewer such superficial problems and, although the people were generally healthy, disease, when it came, tended to be more serious, affecting the inner balance of the *Zang Fu* organs, so herbs – or, as the Yellow Emperor termed them, "poison medicines" – were the preferred choice.

In the cold north of China, practitioners developed moxabustion as a means of warming chilled meridians. In the south, the needle bundle of plum blossom therapy was the preferred method for influencing energy flows. These developed because health problems in this region were likely to be associated with "contracted muscles and numbness."

Massage therapies, including acupressure, and exercise treatments such as *Qigong*, belong historically to central China, where "paralysis, chills, and fevers" were the most common ailments.

CUPPING

Cupping was a familiar treatment to European physicians of up to two hundred years ago, and had been used in the West, as in China, for centuries. The aim is to move or stimulate *Qi* or Blood flow and clear local stagnation by creating a partial vacuum in small glass cups placed on the body. This then "sucks" Blood and fluids through the skin to fill the space.

Cupping is also used to clear external pathogenic evils such as

BELOW **Cupping is used primarily to stimulate *Qi* or Blood flow and clear stagnation.**

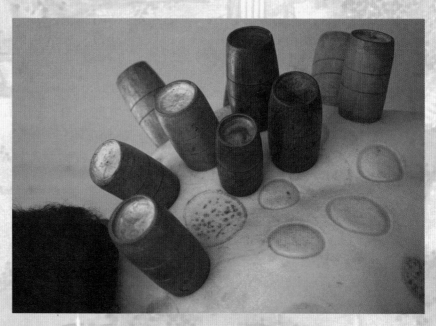

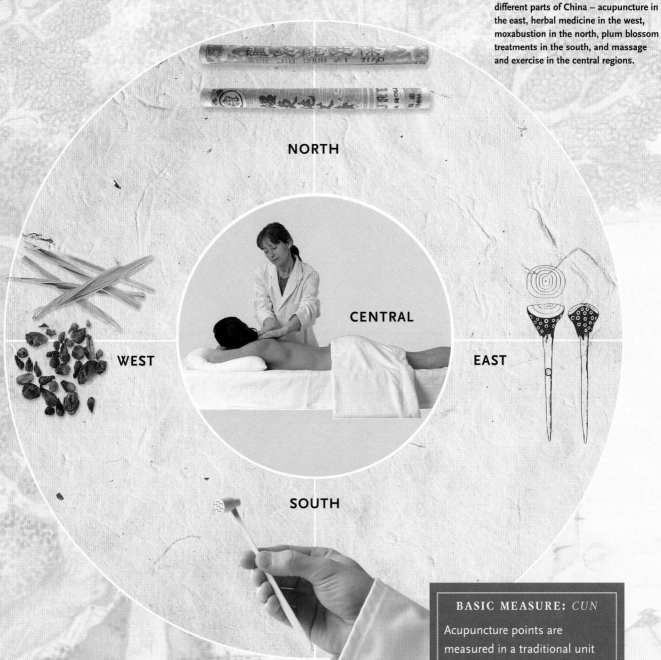

NORTH

WEST

CENTRAL

EAST

SOUTH

Wind–Cold. For this, a large number of cups may be placed over the chest, for example, to help with a respiratory problem.

The practitioner creates the necessary partial vacuum in the cup by burning a small taper inside it to exhaust the oxygen and then placing the cup quickly on the patient's body. The strength of the vacuum varies, depending on how long the taper is burned in the cup, how quickly the cup is placed on the patient, and for how long it is allowed to remain there. Cups may be left in place for only a few seconds or they could be left for some considerable time. Lengthy cupping can result in local weals and bruises that can be quite painful.

BASIC MEASURE: *CUN*

Acupuncture points are measured in a traditional unit called the *cun*, which is the width of the patient's – not the practitioner's – thumb. Basing points location on the patient's *cun* obviously keeps point location in the correct proportion. One-and-a-half *cun* are equivalent to two fingers' width, and three *cun* to four fingers' width.

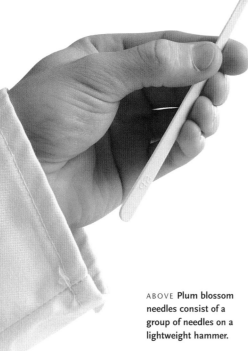

ABOVE **Plum blossom needles consist of a group of needles on a lightweight hammer.**

PLUM BLOSSOM NEEDLE THERAPY

Plum blossom needle therapy originated, according to tradition, in Southern China in the days before the Yellow Emperor. The treatment developed from the shallow insertion of multiple needles at an acu point – a technique variously described in old texts as "superficial needling" or "quick shallow needling."

The "plum blossom needles" used today comprise a handle with a special head for inlaying the needles, and a needle bundle, which is a disc fixed with seven needles. These are usually made of stainless steel around 2.5 cm (1 in) long, although one textbook produced in China in the impoverished 1980s adds that "sewing needles Nos 5–6 will do as well," adding that a bamboo chopstick also makes a perfectly adequate improvized handle.

To give plum blossom needle treatment, the practitioner must hold the handle in his or her right hand at the end, between the middle finger and thumb, with the index finger pressing the middle section. The needle is moved by flexing the wrist to give a regular tap-tap on the acu point.

The tapping may be:
• light – which is considered to be "reinforcing"
• heavy – regarded as "reducing," which will cause red spots on the skin and draw a little blood, or
• "moderate," which is both reducing and reinforcing. Treatment may range from a few taps, to prolonged tapping for several minutes.

Plum blossom needle therapy is used for a wide range of ailments. Tapping on the *Yintang* point (*see* page 120), for example, is used for headaches or facial paralysis, while tapping systematically along both sides of the spinal column is used for sunstroke or feverish colds.

RIGHT **In *Qigong* massage, the therapist uses his or her own vital energy to invigorate the patient.**

MASSAGE

There are a great many different massage techniques used in China. Some are linked to energy stimulating therapies such as *Qigong*, where the practitioner uses his or her own powerful *Qi* to stimulate the patient.

Massage therapy is also used to restore yin–yang balance. Gentle manipulation and stroking are used in deficiency syndromes to restore balance, while, in excess syndromes, heavy manipulation is used to inhibit and reduce the surfeit.

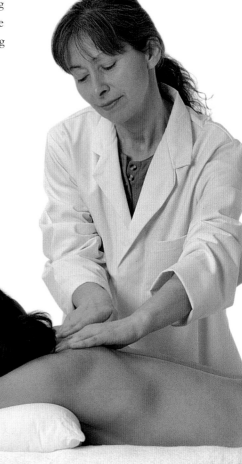

Massage techniques may be divided into eight categories – four yang treatments and four yin. Yang massage includes energetic pushing, pressing, pounding, and knocking techniques, while yin focuses on stroking, smoothing, lifting limbs, or kneading.

Yang treatments are used mainly to clear edema and swellings, reduce pain associated with stagnation, and insomnia. Yin treatments are mainly used for *Qi* and Blood deficiency, general debility and weakness or numbness linked with cold and damp.

EXERCISE

Anyone who has ever visited China will be familiar with the daily exercise rituals that are still followed in many traditional areas. Techniques such as *Qigong* and *t'ai-chi* (*see* pages 130–141) have been used for centuries to improve health and combat disease. Exercise styles vary enormously and are often highly regionalized. The aim is usually to strengthen and simulate the *Qi*, with different exercises focusing on different parts of the body. Some of these can be extremely vigorous, others apparently involving no more than strolling in the park, while slowly twisting and flexing the hand and wrist.

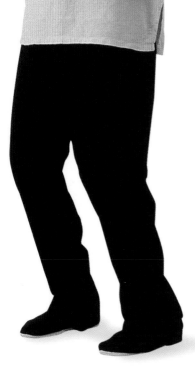

RIGHT *Qigong* and *t'ai-chi* are still everyday routines for many Chinese.

FOUR YANG MASSAGE TECHNIQUES

Technique	Typical methods
Pushing and swaying	pushing, shaking, shifting, holding up, stroking upward
Scattering	pressing lightly, clutching, squeezing, digging
Comforting	stroking, rubbing, scratching, pressing heavily
Pounding and knocking	pounding, thumping, patting, beating

FOUR YIN MASSAGE TECHNIQUES

Technique	Typical methods
Linking and dredging	scrubbing, smoothing, wiping, pressing slightly
Reinforcing *Qi*	trembling, vibrating, tugging, supporting
Kneading and pinching	holding on, holding in, rolling to and fro, kneading
Reconciling collaterals	embracing, stretching, clasping, dragging

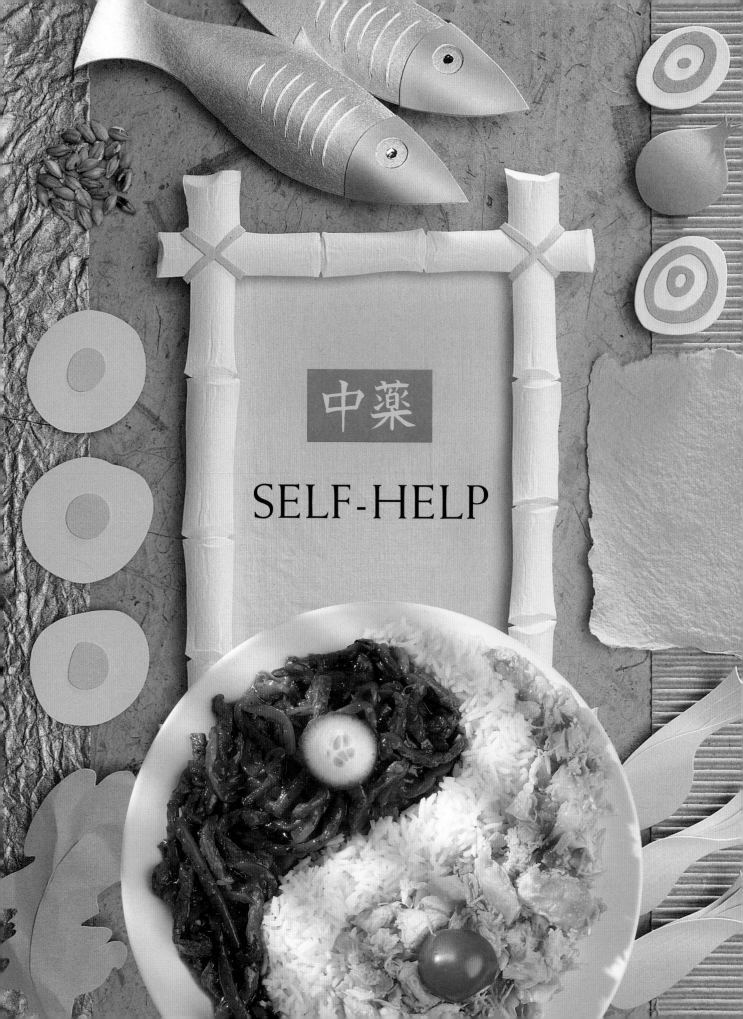

中薬

SELF-HELP

EATING YOUR WAY TO HEALTH

E*ating the right food is central to the Chinese approach to preventive medicine. Balancing the various tastes and characteristics of different foods helps to maintain the inner yin–yang harmony in the individual and so preserve health.*

MAINTAINING BALANCE

In Western terminology, a "healthy diet" usually means one that is rich in the right sorts of nutrients, with plenty of vitamins and minerals, not too much animal fat or sugar, lots of fiber to keep the bowels working, and so forth. The idea that the food needs to reflect one's inner energy demands, or must balance the effects that the changing seasons have on our bodies, is not something which most Westerners consider.

It was not always so. Back in the days of Hippocrates in ancient Greece, food was classified in a similar way to herbs – in terms of their heating and drying qualities. As late as the 17th century the English herbalist

Nicholas Culpeper could happily assume that his readers understood why it was important to eat fennel with fish without the need for a lengthy explanation.

Fish, as we now need to be reminded, is cold and damp, so too much may cause a chill in the stomach. This can be prevented by neutralizing the coldness and dampness of the fish with a hot, dry herb – such as fennel.

CHANGING CHARACTER

As with all things, the Chinese see food in terms of yin and yang balance. Some foods are yin, tending toward cold and dampness, while others are more yang – that is, hot and dry.

Just as Culpeper regarded fish as cold and damp, so the Chinese classify crab as a yin food. Eating too much would make the body more yin, so to combat the imbalance that this could cause, a Chinese cook will always add a pinch of *Zu Si Ye* (purple perilla leaf) to the dish. Just like fennel, this is a warm and pungent herb. Without it a very yin individual would be likely to suffer from diarrhea and stomach cramps due to the cold crab, but, with it, the food is quite safe. A glass of wine – also warming – taken with the crab dish would have a similar effect.

TIME FOR FOOD

The Chinese focus on different sorts of foods at different times of year to reflect the changing yin–yang balance of the seasons (*see* page 109). As well as eating good quality foods in the right season, a healthy diet should include regular, moderate meals. You should never eat to full capacity. The Chinese traditionally eat breakfast – usually a rice or noodle dish with steamed buns – at 6 am, lunch at 12 noon, and evening meal at 6 pm. Between these, there may be snacks of rice noodles or *dim sum* – tasty nibbles like Western *hors d'oeuvres*.

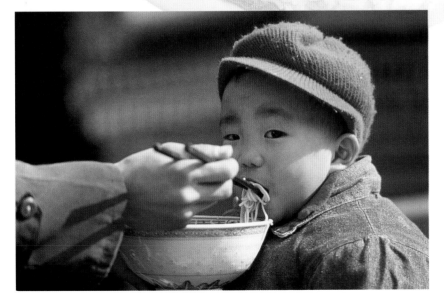

RIGHT **A healthy diet in China consists of regular, moderate meals, including snacks of rice noodles.**

STIMULATING YANG FOODS

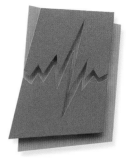

Yang foods should be eaten in winter and only in moderation in the summer, as they are warming. The actual temperature at which food is served does not change its intrinsic qualities significantly, but cooking and storage methods can have important effects.

BLACK TEA

Black tea is made by first wilting the young tips of the tea bush (*Camellia sinensis*) and then fully fermenting them. It is regarded as heating and stimulating and is drunk, without milk, in winter. Brown sugar is also warming, so use it to sweeten your tea on cold days. Unfermented green tea is regarded as more cooling and is the preferred drink in summer.

BUTTER

Butter is warm, sweet and yang, helps to strengthen *Qi* and Blood, and expels any cold. Hot buttered toast with a sprinkling of powdered cinnamon (*see Gui Zhi*, page 67) is a traditional Western treat for winter teatimes. The Chinese regard wheat as cooling, but rye is neutral, so make your winter toast from rye bread instead.

CHICKEN

Chicken is a warm, sweet, yang food that helps to combat cold, strengthen *Qi*, tonify *Jing*, and warm the Middle *Jiao*. It is used in many therapeutic dishes throughout China. Traditionally, after childbirth, it is made into a soup with *Dang Gui* and eaten as a stimulating food. Avoid chicken salads on hot, sunny days, but stir-fry plenty with soy sauce or a pinch of cayenne in winter. Chicken liver is also warming; use it in winter pâtés.

Chicken stir-fry

Herring baked in oatmeal

HERRING

While many fish are regarded as cooling, others are neutral and more stimulating. Herring comes into this category so is an ideal yang food for winter. Roll your herring fillet in beaten egg (neutral), cover with oatmeal (also warming), and bake in the oven for a warming supper dish. Herring is an oily fish and helps to combat dryness and tonify any deficiency. It warms the Middle *Jiao* and is a good supportive food in convalescence.

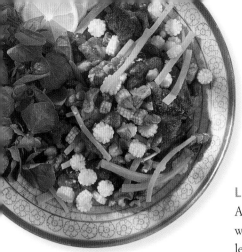

Lamb stir-fry

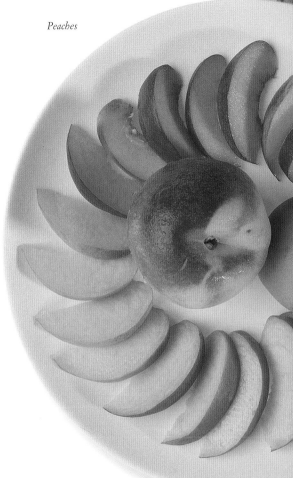

Peaches

LAMB

Lamb and lamb's kidneys are both yang foods, although some Chinese regard the kidneys as rather more warming than the meat. They are good to combat damp and chills, and help to strengthen yang, *Qi*, and Blood. Lamb's kidneys are also believed – in Doctrine of Signatures fashion, whereby a plant's properties are indicated by its appearance – to help the Kidneys, so are recommended for tinnitus, deafness, impotence, or urinary problems, which are all associated with Kidney energy. Lamb itself is seen as more warming for the Stomach and Spleen – useful for diarrhea and stomach chills.

LEEKS AND ONIONS

All members of the *Allium* family are warming, onions rather more so than leeks. Both are regarded as yang, and help to stimulate *Qi* and move congealed Blood. Leeks are often recommended for people suffering from diarrhea, while onions are good for colds, watery nasal catarrh, and stomach chills. Onion soup is an ideal winter warmer, as are stir-fried sliced baby leeks with chicken or thinly cut slices of lamb fillet.

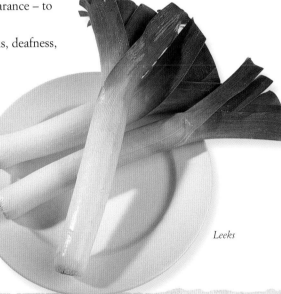

Leeks

PEACHES

Although most fruits are more yin in character, peaches have a tendency to yang. They are warming and stimulating, and will tonify Blood and *Qi*, helping to expel cold and lubricate the system. The seeds are used in herbal medicine, while the fruits are important in food therapy. Duck (neutral) can be made into a warm winter dish by serving it with slices of peach or a peach sauce. An excess of peaches can be damaging; eating too many peaches in summer could lead to Internal Heat syndrome. Cool your peaches with home-made ice cream and raspberry coulis, as in a peach Melba, when the weather is very hot. Apricots, although very similar to peaches, are more neutral in temperature.

WARM AND HOT FOODS AND SUBSTANCES

Warm foods or substances	brown sugar, cherry, chicken, chives, dates, scallions, ham, kumquat, leek, mutton, peach, raspberry, prawns, walnuts, wine, tobacco, sunflower seeds
Hot foods	pepper, ginger, green and red peppers, soybean oil

101

CALMING YIN FOODS

*Y*in foods should be eaten in summer and only in moderation in the winter, as they are all very cooling. Storing food in a freezer is believed by some to make food even cooler and heavier, and can affect the intrinsic nature of certain dishes.

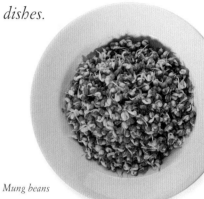

Mung beans

BROAD BEANS

Like many beans, broad beans tend toward coldness and damp with a yin character. They're sometimes used as a Spleen tonic and can help diarrhea. Broad beans are an ideal summer vegetable – tossed in butter on cooler days or warmed with a little mint if you find their cold, damp nature leads to flatulence!

MUNG BEANS

Sprouted mung beans are the bean sprouts of popular Westernized Chinese cookery, which are regularly added to stir-fries and mixed vegetable dishes. They are sweet and cold, tending toward yin. They can help to clear heat from the system, tonify *Qi* and Blood, and strengthen yin. They should be avoided in cases of yang deficiency; otherwise, eat plenty in summer salads.

Banana split

BANANA

Bananas are cold, *yin*, and sweet, and will tonify *Qi* and Blood. They are commonly used for constipation and help to lubricate the Intestines. They're the ideal food for hot summer days. Serve banana splits with home-made sorbet or ice cream.

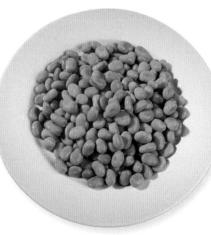

Broad beans

CRAB

Crab is cold, salty, and yin. It can clear heat and is an excellent yin tonic. Crabs are good summer eating, but may need the help of a pinch of purple perilla in fall, or if those eating them have any sort of yang deficiency or problems with Wind. In Chinese folk medicine, crab is believed to help reconnect fractured bones, and is also used to combat burns and irritant heat rashes.

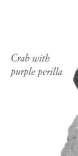

Crab with purple perilla

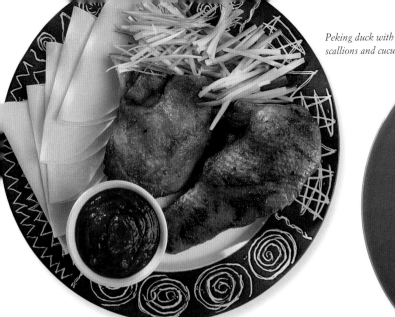

*Peking duck with
scallions and cucumber*

Beancurd stew

DUCK

Duck is sweet, neutral to cool and tending toward yin. It is often eaten when there is any sort of Hot syndrome, fevers, coughs, or swellings, for example, and is believed to nourish the Stomach. Duck is a good summer food and provides a calming interlude in a long banquet. It is no surprise that "Peking duck" is traditionally served as the second or third course of a long meal in order to calm and nourish the stomach, ready for the labors ahead. The slivers of cucumber (cool) and scallion (warm) served with Peking duck allow diners to warm or cool the dish to meet their own needs.

LETTUCE

Lettuce is cool, slightly bitter and tending toward yin. It helps to calm overexuberant yang and is also drying, making it ideal for Damp–Heat syndromes. It is a diuretic and is used in China for urinary problems – especially oliguria (scanty urination). Lettuce is a traditional accompaniment to peas in French cooking and it is a good pairing. Peas are yang and warming, so adding lettuce helps to cool the dish and maintain well-being. Lettuce also affects the Stomach and Large Intestine, so can be a good digestive remedy for the start of a meal.

BEANCURD/TOFU

Beancurd, made from soya beans, is – like the beans themselves – cooling and tonifying for yin. It is a good *Qi* and Blood food, helping to clear Heat and encourage Body Fluids. Beancurd stews and casseroles are summer favorites in many parts of southern China. Cook with broad beans or pork for a more yin meal or add lamb and carrots for a yang dish.

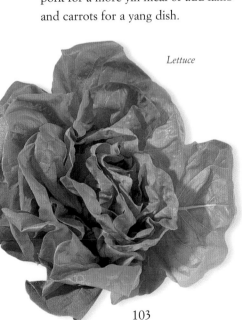

Lettuce

COLD, COOL, AND NEUTRAL FOODS

Cold foods
bamboo shoots, banana, clams, crab, grapefruit, lettuce, persimmon, seaweed, star fruit, water chestnut, watercress, watermelon

Cool foods
tomato, apple, barley, beancurd, button mushrooms, cucumber, lettuce, mango, mung beans, pear, spinach, strawberry

Neutral foods
apricot, beef, beetroot, Chinese leaves, carrot, celery, egg, corn (maize), honey, polished white rice, potato, pumpkin, white sugar

TASTY DISHES

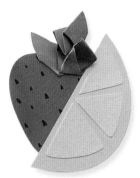

*J*ust *as the taste of herbs indicates the organs that they will affect, according to the five-element theory, so the taste of food is also a therapeutic indicator. Mixing different tastes at a meal is important to maintain overall balance between the organs.*

ALL SORTS OF FLAVORS

As well as the five major tastes of pungent, sweet, sour, bitter, and salty, food – like herbs – may also be astringent or bland (also described as neutral). Astringent and sour tastes are very similar, so it is easiest to combine these together to give six distinct flavors. Like herbs, different tasting foods have a specific effect on the body.

Pungent foods – which can also be thought of as "spicy" – are defined as "dispersing and flowing." These foods help to remove toxins from the system and stimulate the circulation of *Qi* and Blood. Pungent is the flavor also associated by Chinese physicians with the Lungs, Large Intestine, nose, and sense of smell.

Sweet tastes are very nutritious, warming, and tonifying. Just as many Chinese tonic herbs, such as *Ren Shen*, have a sweet taste, so too do many starchy cereals and sugar, which explains why a cake or biscuit can sometimes be comforting. Sweet is the taste associated with the Spleen and Stomach.

Sour tastes are astringent and absorbent, and "tighten" tissues – an effect rather like using aftershave or a toner on the skin. Sour foods can

often be helpful for problems like diarrhea, while the sour taste is associated with the Liver.

Bitter tastes are described as "drying and purging," and will stimulate digestive function. Bitter is associated with the Heart.

Salty flavors are associated with Water and the Kidneys, and are defined as "softening and descending." Salty herbs are

used to disperse hard swellings, and salty foods can be useful as lubricants to help disperse toxic accumulations in the body.

Neutral foods tend to be diuretic to encourage urination. They also help the body rid itself of unwanted toxins. Sweet, pungent, and neutral flavors tend to be more yang, while salty, bitter, and sour flavors are more yin.

RIGHT **Meal of different tastes: asparagus (bitter); fennel (pungent); pork (salty); and tomato (sour).**

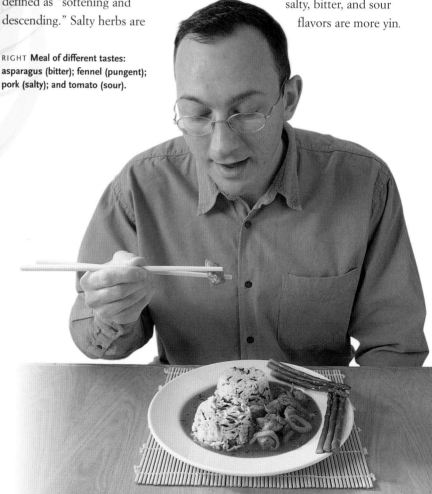

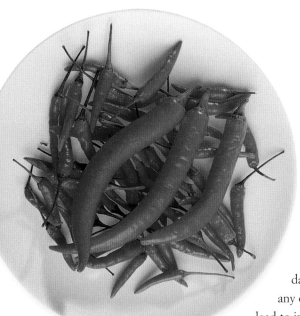

ABOVE **Too much spicy food, such as chilies, may damage the *Qi* and Blood, and may lead to yin deficiency.**

NOTHING TO EXCESS

The different tastes of food can have a positive effect on the *Zang Fu* organs and fundamental substances (*see* pages 14–27), but they can also be damaging. An excess of any of the flavors is likely to lead to imbalance and poor health. Too much hot, spicy food, for example, could potentially damage the *Qi* and Blood, and possibly result in yin deficiency.

Too many sweet foods – as is common in many Western diets – can lead to overdominance of the Spleen and Stomach, which, in turn, following the five-element model, may overcontrol Water and damage Kidney *Qi*. Sweet foods are yang and heating, so can lead to excess Fire, which could attack the Heart as well. In Western terms, too many sweets and sugars may lead to obesity or high cholesterol levels, which could cause atherosclerosis and coronary heart disease. In Chinese terms, excess Heat is to blame for damaging the Heart, but the end result is very similar.

THE TASTES OF SOME COMMON FOODS AND SUBSTANCES

Pungent foods or substances	red and green peppers, tobacco, soybean oil, garlic, fennel, kumquat, rice bran, wine, pepper, leek, scallions, sweet basil, chives, ginger, wine
Sweet foods	ripe fruits (including apples, banana, dates, oranges, grapes, pineapple), eggplant, beancurd, bamboo shoots, beef, beetroot, butter, button mushrooms, carrots, celery, cherries, coffee, Chinese leaves, Chinese black fungus, broad beans, chicken, chicken eggs, cucumber, sweet potatoes, honey, wheat, sugar, shiitake mushroom, mung beans, mango, lettuce, peanuts, pumpkin, lamb's kidney, chicken livers, lamb's liver, calves' liver, cow's milk, pork, shrimps, wine
Sour foods	lemon, unripe fruits (such as apple, pear, grapefruit, plum, tomato, mango), vinegar, duck, olives
Bitter foods	asparagus, lettuce, coffee, hops, pumpkin, lamb's liver, vinegar, wine
Salty foods	seaweed, salt, chive seeds, duck, ham, oysters, clams, crab, barley, pig's kidney, pork

NB: *Some foods have more than one flavor.*

Meal of varied tastes

HEALTHY MENUS

*C*hoosing the right tastes is a simple way to help combat any inbuilt tendencies in Zang Fu *or energy balance. Choosing the right flavors makes simple – and delicious – preventive medicine.*

FOODS TO STRENGTHEN SPLEEN *Qi*

Deficient Spleen or Stomach *Qi* and Spleen yang deficiency are common syndromes in the West, and are usually characterized by poor appetite, abdominal bloating and discomfort, tiredness, and a tendency to loose stools or diarrhea. Typically, the tongue is pale with a white coating, and the pulse is weak. It is the sort of problem that might be labeled as "irritable bowel syndrome" in Western medicine and can also be associated with nervous indigestion or a tendency to gastric ulcers.

Eating plenty of sweet foods will help to restore balance to the system, so the diet should be rich in foods like cooked carrots, sweet potatoes, turnips, leeks, onions, sweet rice, butter, lamb, chicken, cooked peaches, honey, maple syrup, and sugar. Foods to avoid include salads, citrus fruit, salt, dairy products, and too much liquid taken with meals.

Cold or raw foods should be avoided, as bringing them up to body temperature once they've been swallowed simply expends more Stomach energy. In Tibetan medicine, it is considered that freezing food also changes its character, making it colder – not so much a problem with food that has been frozen when raw, but possibly damaging with frozen prepared meals, since their character has been changed in cooking. It is thought that freezing leftovers for use in a later meal can chill them, leading to an increased risk of damaging Spleen and Stomach *Qi*.

A suitable dish for Spleen *Qi* deficiency could be:

COOKING TIP
Start the meal with a bowl of onion soup, and finish with sliced peaches cooked in the oven with a little wine and honey

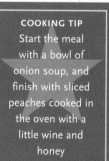

RIGHT **Stir-fried beef with plain rice would be a suitable dish for those suffering from weak Spleen *Qi*.**

BEEF STIR-FRY

1 lb (c.500 g) beef fillet pieces, cut into thin strips
5 oz (125 g) finely sliced baby leeks
5 oz (125 g) finely sliced baby carrots
1 clove garlic crushed
1 teaspoon chopped fresh ginger
1 dessertspoon of olive oil
1 tablespoon of seasoned flour
1 small glass red wine
1 teaspoon tomato purée
$1/4$ pint (150 ml) of beef or chicken stock
salt, pepper, and a pinch of sugar

Sauté the carrots and leeks in the olive oil until they start to soften. Ideally, Chinese therapeutic meals should be cooked with as little oil as possible. If you have a non-stick pan, it is usually possible to dry-fry meats, although vegetables may need a little oil to improve the cooking. Toss the beef slices in the seasoned flour, then add to the pan with the garlic and ginger. Cook for about five minutes until the meat is browned, add the red wine and bubble vigorously for a couple of minutes, then add the stock and tomato purée. Season and serve on a bed of plain boiled rice. Thin slices of lamb fillet can be used instead of beef, if you prefer.

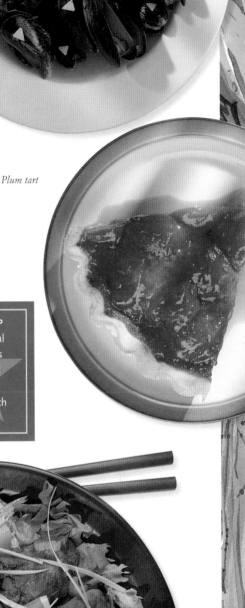

Mussels in garlic
and white wine

FOODS TO CONTROL
EXCESS LIVER *QI*

Overexuberant Liver *Qi* is another
common syndrome. It is typified by
emotional instability – irritability or
anger, a sensation of a lump in the
throat, or problems swallowing, lumps
in the neck, groin, or breast (including
benign fibrocystitis). The tongue is
usually a darkish purple or brown,
and the pulse is wiry.

Disorders typically seen in the West
that may come into the excess Liver
Qi category include premenstrual
syndrome, depression, as well
as dysmenorrhea.

Foods that may aggravate the Liver
or add to the excess *Qi* include any
that are sour tasting, and foods that
contain toxins or chemicals that are
difficult to digest. The Liver is the
body's first line of defense, taking the
products of digestion, checking they
are not harmful, and adding them to
the Blood system. Toxic chemicals
tend to remain "stuck" in the liver;
both Western and Chinese herbalists
regularly talk of the "Liver stagnation"
that these pollutants cause.

Foods to stimulate *Qi* and improve
its flow are also important, so the diet
should contain some pungent flavors –
such as basil, ginger, or garlic –
although these should be used in
moderation, as an excess could be
damaging. Foods to relax the liver
are also helpful – e.g., dishes
containing chicken livers, celery,
mussels, or plums.

A suitable dish for excess Liver *Qi*
would be:

CHICKEN LIVERS
AND MANGO

*1 lb (c.500 g) fresh chicken livers,
cut into bite-size pieces*

1–2 tablespoons of seasoned flour

*1 small, ripe mango, peeled and
cut into cubes*

1 dessertspoon of olive oil

1 tablespoon of balsamic vinegar

salt and freshly ground black pepper

Toss the chicken livers in seasoned flour
so that they are well coated. Stir-fry
them in the olive oil for five
minutes until they are
browned on the outside but
not overcooked. Add the
balsamic vinegar, and let it
bubble for a minute, then
remove from the heat, add
the mango, and mix well.
Serve on a bed of lettuce with
a little shredded celery and
baby leeks added.

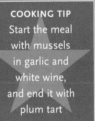

COOKING TIP
Start the meal
with mussels
in garlic and
white wine,
and end it with
plum tart

Plum tart

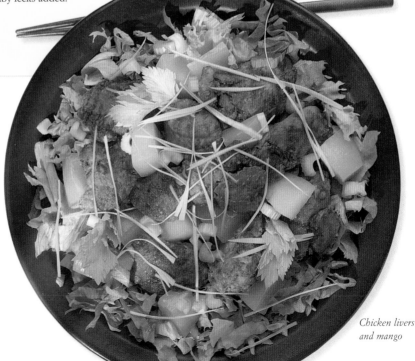

Chicken livers
and mango

FOOD TO STRENGTHEN *WEI QI*

In Western terms, deficient *Wei Qi* would be equated with a weakened immune system. If *Wei Qi* is weak, then exogenous pathogens can easily enter and damage the body, and the result would be recurrent chills, colds, chest infections, or sore throats, as well as a tendency for allergic reactions. Sufferers are often tired, feel the cold easily, and have a general pallor and lack of energy.

Warming foods to tonify the *Qi* and strengthen the Lungs are needed. This could include the use of tonic herbs like *Ren Shen*, *Dang Shen*, and *Huang Qi*, which may be added to stews, soups, and casseroles. Plenty of nutritious vegetables and well-cooked grains will help, but salty foods should be avoided, as they send the *Qi* downward, and *Wei Qi* needs to flow out and onto the surface. A downward action could thus damage it still further.

Onions and garlic are especially good for strengthening the *Wei Qi*, or try this warming chicken dish:

Mixed vegetables side dish

CHICKEN WITH *HUANG QI* AND SHIITAKE MUSHROOMS

1 chicken – jointed into six pieces in the usual way with the carcass
approx. 1¾ pints (1 liter) of water
2 thin slices of Huang Qi (*milk vetch*)
salt and pepper
1 dessertspoon of olive oil
9 oz (250 g) shiitake mushrooms, sliced
1 teaspoon finely chopped ginger
1 clove garlic, finely sliced

Put the chicken carcass into a slow cooker, cover with boiling water, add the *Huang Qi,* and cook overnight.

Alternatively, cook in the oven (270°F/140°C/Gas mark 1) for at least three hours, or simmer the pot on the lowest setting on the hob. Make sure your pot has a well-fitting lid so that the chicken will not dry out.

When the stock is ready, strain off the liquid and set aside. Rub the chicken pieces with salt and pepper, and place them in a shallow roasting pot in the oven (400°F/200°C/Gas mark 6) for 30 minutes. Meanwhile, stir-fry the shiitake mushrooms in olive oil with the garlic and ginger until they have softened. Add this to the strained chicken stock.

Pour off any surplus fat from the chicken dish and then pour over the shiitake and stock mixture and baste well. Return to the oven for 25 minutes, basting regularly. Remove the *Huang Qi* before serving, as it is too fibrous to eat.

Serve with French bread croutons and mixed vegetables as a side dish.

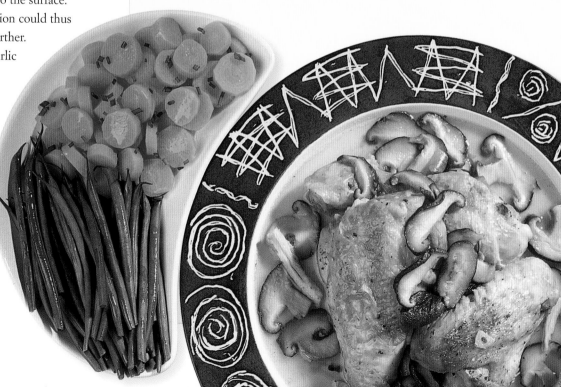

Leek soup

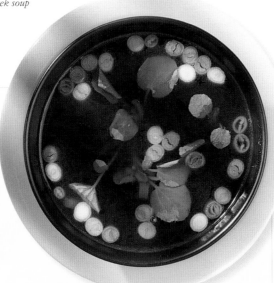

> **COOKING TIP**
> Start the meal
> with leek or
> onion soup
> and finish with
> an apple and
> blackberry tart

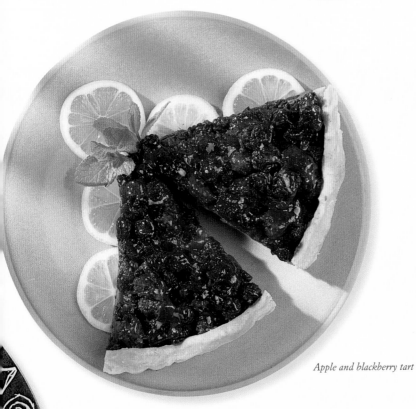

Apple and blackberry tart

Chicken with Huang Qi
and shiitake mushrooms

SEASONAL DELIGHTS

SPRING
Neutral food is needed –
the weather tends to be
changeable, and so a
balance of yin and yang
dishes is needed to help
the body cope with sudden
changes in climate. Dishes
should be neither
predominantly cooling nor
overstimulating.

SUMMER
This is a very yang time, so
cooling meals are needed
to support yin. Less meat
with more vegetables and
fish dishes are ideal. Oily,
fatty foods should also be
avoided and alcoholic
intake should be limited, as
this is heating.

FALL
The weather starts to
become more yin again, so
warmer dishes are needed:
more meat and a little less
of the very yin fruits.

WINTER
The weather is cold
and so is the body – yin
dominates and it is time
for heating foods: more
alcohol, and hot meats
such as lamb and chicken
rather than pork and duck,
which are slightly cooler.

THERAPEUTIC RICE DISHES

*C*hinese families make a variety of therapeutic rice dishes for treating minor household ills or to support prescribed herbal remedies. They're usually called congee *by Westerners after the Anglo-Indian* word for porridge, *but the Chinese call them* Shi-fan *(water rice).*

COOKING *CONGEE*

Congee is a sort of thin rice gruel which can easily be made by putting a cup of rice with six cups of water in a heavy-bottomed, lidded saucepan.

Set the pot on the lowest possible heat on the hob and simmer for up to six hours. Stir the pot regularly to prevent the congee from sticking. Alternatively, use a slow cooker and leave the mixture overnight – this is ideal if you are making *congee* for breakfast. Stir the mixture as soon as you can in the morning.

Plain *congee* is often served for breakfast in parts of China with an assortment of side dishes, such as hard-boiled eggs or steamed buns.

A very wide range of other ingredients can also be added to the rice mix to create a variety of therapeutic meals.

VARIANTS ON A THEME

Congee can be cooked with medicinal herbs – such as *Shu Di Huang* or *Gou Qi Zi* – as an alternative to the usual *tangs* or soups. The herbs are put into the pot about halfway through cooking.

An alternative tradition is to follow a bowl of herbal *tang* with a bowl of congee. This provides a second supportive medicinal effect.

In some Chinese herbal restaurants, an assortment of *congees* may be on offer. Each dish is designed specifically to help a particular type of ailment: additional ingredients like shrimp, chicken livers, kidneys, peas, or bamboo shoots turn the *congee* into a complete meal.

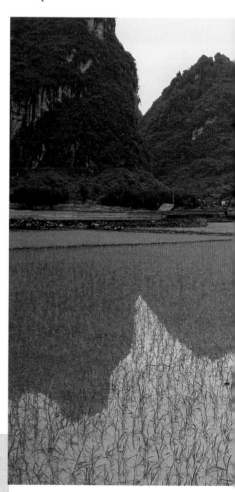

RIGHT **In Buddhist tradition**, *congee* **made with milk and honey was seen as a preventative against poor health.**

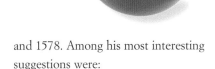

For breakfast, a popular *congee* contains Chinese red dates, fresh ginger, and honey. Ginger is pungent so helps *Qi* and Blood circulation. The red dates are calming for *Shen* (spirit), and the honey helps to lubricate the digestive system and nourish the Heart – a good way to start the day.

Note that rice is a diuretic, so *congee* needs to be avoided in cases of Kidney *Qi* or Kidney yang deficiency.

BELOW **Rice is not only China's staple food, it also acts as a herbal remedy in the form of *congee*.**

PORRIDGE POTIONS

Congees have been recommended for a range of ailments since ancient times. In Buddhist tradition, *congee* made with milk and honey was regarded as a general preventive against poor health. It was said to confer "life, beauty, ease, and strength," and would dispel "hunger, thirst, and wind," as well as help digestion and "cleanse the bladder."

The 16th-century herbalist Li Shi Zhen recommended a variety of congees in his great herbal, the **Ben Cao Gang Mu**, written between 1552 and 1578. Among his most interesting suggestions were:

• wheat *congee* – believed to be cooling and calming with a nourishing effect on the Heart
• chestnut *congee* – which will help to tonify the Kidneys and strengthen the lower back
• radish *congee* – a digestive tonic to cool the system
• ginger *congee* – with dried ginger added to the mix to combat Cold and deficiency problems that may lead to indigestion and diarrhea
• liver *congee* – with chopped liver added to the mixture as a remedy for Liver deficiency syndromes
• aduki bean *congee* – aduki beans are sometimes called "red dragon beans" and are a tonic food for the Kidneys; this congee is used to help with fluid retention and urinary dysfunction
• leek or onion *congee* – used as a warming remedy for the digestive system, suitable in cases of diarrhea
• apricot seed *congee* – used as an expectorant for chest problems, including productive coughs and asthma.

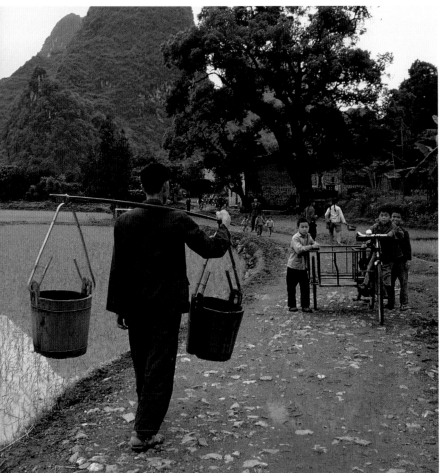

TONIC WINES

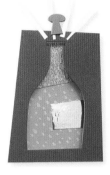

onic wines are an easy way to make and take healing herbs. Many use a single herb, although traditional combinations aimed at specific organs and energy problems can also be produced at home. Here is a simple guide to making your own tonic wines at home.

MAKING TONIC WINES

The simplest way to make a tonic wine is to use a vinegar vat – a crock pot holding 3–5 pints (2–3 liters) with an open top, closed with a large cork, and a small tap at the bottom. They can be bought from cook stores, home-brewing specialists or craft potters. A vinegar vat is ideal, as the tonic wine can be drawn off from the bottom, while a fresh supply of wine is easy to add at the top. You can make tonic wines in any glass jar, but strain the mixture before use.

Fill the vat with the herb or herb mixture. Cover with wine (red or white) and leave for at least two weeks, although four to eight weeks is generally better. It is important to cover the herb completely; otherwise, it will go moldy and have to be discarded. Draw a daily sherry glass dose of your brew from the tap and fill the container with additional wine so as to keep the herb covered. This sort of vat can be used for months.

If you are using a glass jar, put 9 oz (250 g) of herb (if using root herbs) into the jar and cover it with wine (about two cups). Shake well and, after two to eight weeks, strain the mix through a muslin bag, wine press, or nylon strainer. Bottle in clean glass bottles and use in sherry-glass doses.

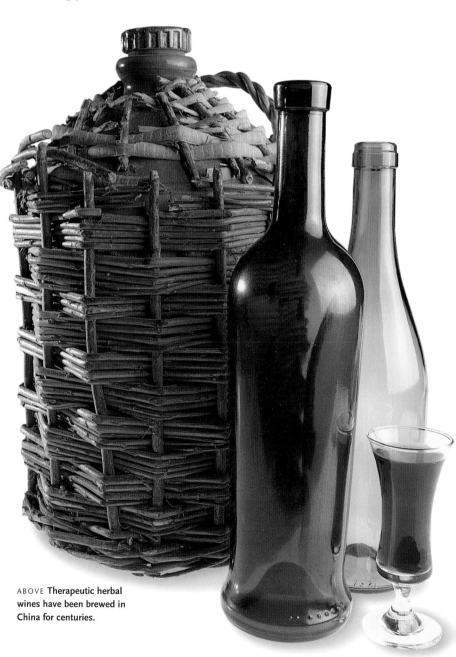

ABOVE **Therapeutic herbal wines have been brewed in China for centuries.**

112

SIMPLE TONIC WINES TO MAKE AT HOME

• *Da Zao Jiu* – made from whole red Chinese dates. Use to replenish Spleen and Stomach *Qi* and to nourish the blood.

• *Dang Gui Jiu* – made from the chopped root. A traditional female tonic to nourish Blood and invigorate the circulation. Combine with half as much *Dan Shen* as a menstrual tonic for period pains and irregular menstruation. A traditional tonic after childbirth is to combine *Dang Gui* with *Bai Shao*, *Wu Wei Zi*, *Shan Yao*, *Du Zhong*, *Gan Cao*, and *Gou Qi Zi.* Use equal amounts of the first four herbs to half as much of the last three. *Dang Shen* – made from the chopped root. Use as a general *Qi* tonic and to stimulate Blood production. Particularly good for the Spleen, Stomach and Lungs, and significantly less expensive than *Ren Shen*.

• *Du Zhong* wine – made from chopped pieces of bark. Use to tonify Kidney and Liver *Qi* and *Jing*; also helpful for back pain associated with Kidney deficiency, and in cases of infertility/impotence.

• *Gou Qi Zi Jiu* – made from the whole berries. Use as a tonic for Liver and Kidney yin and to improve the eyesight. *Caution:* Take only in tablespoon doses, as overconsumption can be damaging. Be sure to buy good-quality herbs; cases of *Gou Qi Zi* contaminated with ephedrine have been recorded.

• *He Shou Wu Jiu* – made from the sliced root. Use as a tonic for Liver and Kidney yin and *Jing,* and to nourish the Blood. This is a traditional longevity remedy that will also help to combat prematurely graying hair.

• *Huang Qi Jiu* – made from the dried root – tonifies yang *Qi* and *Wei Qi*.

• *Ren Shen Huang Qi Jiu* – use twice as much *Huang Qi* as *Ren Shen* to create a strong *Qi* tonic. This is especially useful for Lung weakness or following influenza.

• *Shan Yao Jiu* – made from slices of root. Use as a tonic for Spleen and Stomach to improve digestion, and also to strengthen Kidney and Liver *Qi* and *Jing.*

• Walnut wine – made from shelled nuts or *Hu Tao Ren.* It can be used as a tonic for the Lungs, Kidneys, and *Jing.* It also is used for back pain related to Kidney deficiency, and for respiratory problems.

RIGHT **A sherry glass of tonic every day will help boost your** *Qi.*

PRESSING FOR HEALTH

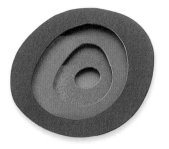

*A*cupressure *("finger pressure") is a self-help technique based on traditional Chinese therapies. The aim is to prevent disease, or, as the Yellow Emperor put it, "…the sages did not treat those who were already ill; they instructed those who were not yet ill."*

ALL SORTS OF MASSAGE

The art of manipulating various acupuncture points to improve energy flows and well-being, is the basis of several Chinese and Japanese therapeutic techniques that have become popular in the West in the past decade.

Acupressure is the basis of Japanese Shiatsu (*shiatsu* also means "finger pressure"), which has developed into a therapy in its own right over the past century. As well as shiatsu*,* the basic acupressure techniques have evolved into numerous styles and go under various names, such as *G-Jo, Jin Shin Do, Wushu,* and *Do-In.*

Acupressure is normally described as "acupuncture without needles," but that is something of an oversimplification for the various techniques that can be involved in the different methods.

Wushu, or "pointing therapy," for example, involves pinching, pressing, patting, and knocking and, as with *Qigong* massage (*see* pages 96–97), practitioners need to be experts in *Qi*-strengthening skills. The prime action or "pointing" involves tapping the acu

point, usually with the middle finger alone, or with the thumb and first two fingers closed together, every two or three seconds for several minutes; at the same time, therapists need to focus their vital energies on their own arm and fingers delivering the treatment. "Pinching" is a technique applied only to fingers, toes, or nails, which is where the major meridians start, while "patting" is used to promote energy and Blood flow, and involves tapping a flat hand five to ten times against various meridians. "Knocking" is very similar, only using four fingers and thumb.

"Pointing" treatments also use pressure from a lightly clenched fist and the second thumb joint (rather than the tip).

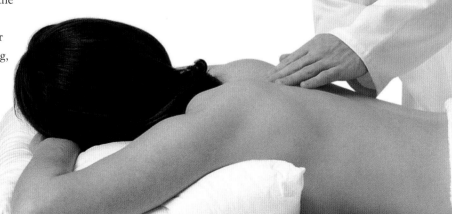

APPLYING PRESSURE

Although it is common in Western interpretations of acupressure to press with the tip of the thumb, the clenched fist action of "pointing therapy" using the second thumb joint can be more comfortable. Others prefer to use the tip of their first or second finger – but remember to keep nails short and always start with gentle pressure until you understand the effects of the action.

Maintain pressure for two to three minutes while focusing as much healing energy as you can into your hands to help boost deficient *Qi* levels. A gentle, rotating motion applied to the point is helpful for dispersing stagnant *Qi* and improving energy flows. Like all Chinese therapies, it is essential for the practitioner to give his or her total concentration during treatment – you cannot practice acupressure effectively if your mind is elsewhere.

LEFT **Acupressure treatments are ideal for both chronic health problems and minor conditions.**

HOW DOES IT WORK?

While the Chinese have simply accepted the effectiveness of acupuncture and acupressure for generations, Western medicine constantly seeks a scientific explanation. Most current theories focus on the production of endorphins.

These are the body's own painkillers and are peptides or protein molecules created from a substance called *beta-lipotropin* found in the pituitary gland. Endorphins are thought to control the activity of the endocrine glands where they are stored, and also affect the pain-sensing areas in the brain in a way very similar to opiate drugs such as morphine.

Endorphin release is controlled by the nervous system. Nerves are, of course, sensitive to pain and outside stimuli, and, once triggered, will instruct the endocrine system to release appropriate endorphins. Pressing acu points is believed to have a similar effect on endorphin production.

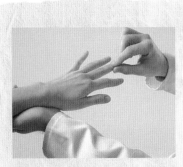

ABOVE **"Pinching" is a technique applied only to fingers, toes or nails, which is where the major meridians start.**

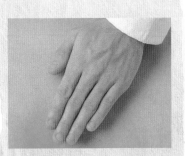

ABOVE **"Patting" is used to promote energy and blood flow and involves tapping a flat hand 5–10 times against various meridians.**

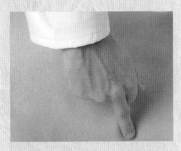

ABOVE **"Pointing" involves tapping the acu point, usually with the middle finger alone or with the thumb and first two fingers closed together, every 2–3 seconds for several minutes.**

ACUPRESSURE IN HOME FIRST AID

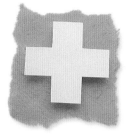

*A*pplying pressure to easily accessible *acu points can offer the ideal home treatment for simple self-limiting disorders and also in home first aid.*

Points on the meridians or energy channels of the body (shown below and opposite) are known as acu points. It is sometimes possible to feel these acu points as tiny nodules under the skin; pressing them will often trigger a sensation or feeling of relief.

Locate the point by touch (if you can) or use the traditional measurement based on the patient's thumb width – the *cun* (*see* page 95). Remember that one-and-a-half *cun* are equivalent to two fingers' width, and three cun to four fingers' width.

Apart from the 361 main points (*see* pages 88–89), there are dozens of extraordinary points. The suggestions given in the following pages of useful acu points for specific illnesses are all reasonably easy to locate.

KEY TO MERIDIANS
—— Lung (LU)
—— Large Intestine (LI)
—— Stomach (ST)
—— Spleen (SP)
—— Heart (HT)
—— Small Intestine (SI)
—— Urinary Bladder (UB)
—— Kidney (KD)
—— Pericardium (PC)
—— San Jiao (SJ)
—— Gall Bladder (GB)
—— Liver (LV)
—— Governing Vessel (GV)
—— Conception Vessel (CV)

CAUTIONS
• Do not apply acupressure to areas of broken or infected skin, sores, or burns.

• Avoid acupressure if someone has a high fever, acute illness, or varicose veins.

• Use only limited acupressure in pregnancy, as overstimulation of certain acu points may lead to miscarriage.

• Do not give acupressure to the very elderly, chronically ill, or those suffering from Heart or Liver diseases. Professional treatment only is recommended.

• Always try acupressure on yourself before you attempt to give it to others so that you have a better understanding of how it feels.

NB: The remedies suggested here are for minor self-limiting problems that could be included in the category of household first aid. If symptoms persist, seek professional help.

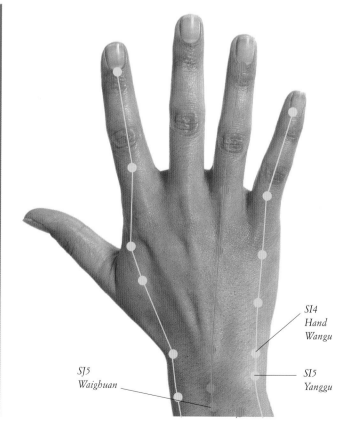

SI4 Hand Wangu

SI5 Yanggu

SJ5 Waighuan

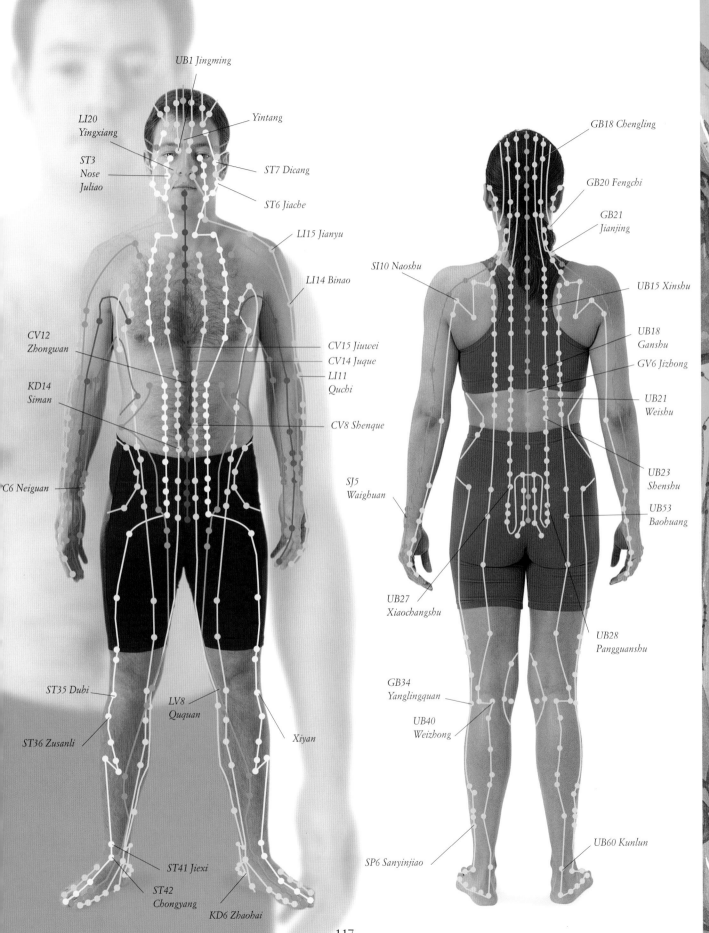

UB1 Jingming

Yintang

LI20 Yingxiang

ST3 Nose Juliao

ST7 Dicang

ST6 Jiache

LI15 Jianyu

LI14 Binao

CV12 Zhongwan

CV15 Jiuwei

CV14 Juque

LI11 Quchi

KD14 Siman

CV8 Shenque

PC6 Neiguan

SJ5 Waighuan

ST35 Dubi

LV8 Ququan

Xiyan

ST36 Zusanli

ST41 Jiexi

ST42 Chongyang

KD6 Zhaohai

GB18 Chengling

GB20 Fengchi

GB21 Jianjing

SI10 Naoshu

UB15 Xinshu

UB18 Ganshu

GV6 Jizhong

UB21 Weishu

UB23 Shenshu

UB53 Baohuang

UB27 Xiaochangshu

UB28 Pangguanshu

GB34 Yanglingquan

UB40 Weizhong

SP6 Sanyinjiao

UB60 Kunlun

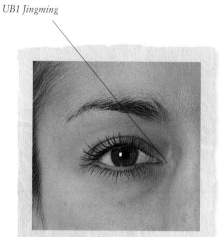

UB1 *Jingming*

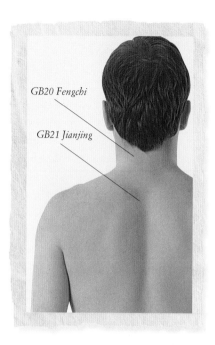

GB20 *Fengchi*

GB21 *Jianjing*

HEADACHE

Several points can be effective for headache. A popular recommendation is the *Yintang* point (one of the extraordinary points), which lies between the eyebrows in the center of the forehead: this is also a good point for helping to clear the mind and improve concentration. Pressure on the *Yintang* point is ideal to help lift the energy levels of desk-bound workers during the afternoon.

Other valuable points for treating headache are:
GB21 (*Jianjing*) – in line with the seventh cervical vertebra, on the trapezium muscle at the base of the neck, slightly behind the highest point on the shoulder. In China, "pointing" **GB21** with a stirring motion is preferred to simple pressure.
LI4 (*Hegu*) – found on the web between the thumb and forefinger,

high up in the valley between the joints. As well as headaches, this point is used for general pain relief and specifically for pains in the wrist and hand.
LV1 (*Dadun*) – where the nail meets the flesh on the inside edge of the big toe. Another convenient point for self-administration – a firm pressure should be applied here for two to three minutes.

MIGRAINE

GB20 (*Fengchi*) – at the base of the skull in a hollow between two bands of muscle. This point is often sensitive to pressure, and also helps to release any sort of neck and head tensions. It is also used for insomnia and dizziness, colds, influenza, neck pains, and nervous problems.

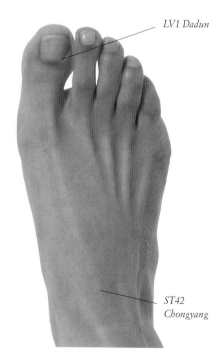

LV1 *Dadun*

ST42 *Chongyang*

TIRED EYES

ST36 (*Zusanli*) – in the hollow outside the shinbone, located two *cun* below the kneecap.
UB1 (*Jingming*) – in the inner corner of the eye. Apply only gentle pressure, because this can be a sensitive area.

TOOTHACHE

Acupressure can provide temporary pain relief until dental treatment is available. **LI14** – on the outer edge of the upper arm, below the deltoid muscle midway between the elbow and shoulder – is generally helpful for a range of tooth problems, while pressing **LI20** (*Yingxiang*) – in the hollow where the nostril meets the cheek – is more specific for problems affecting the upper teeth. For pain in the lower teeth, try:
ST6 (*Jiache*) – above the corner of the jaw, one *cun* toward the nose;
ST7 (*Dicang*) – where the upper and lower jaws meet – a hollow is felt here when the jaws are relaxed and slack;
ST42 (*Chongyang*) – at the highest point of the foot in line with the second and third toes.

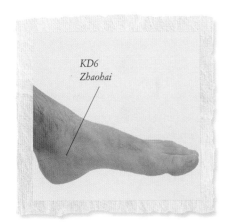

KD6 Zhaohai

EARACHE

KD6 (*Zhaohai*) – this point is directly below the inner ankle bone where there is a small hollow which may be sensitive to pressure. This an important point for Kidney energies and can also help the reproductive organs as well as ease ear pains.

NASAL CONGESTION AND CATARRH

ST3 (*Nose Juliao*) – directly below the eye at the bottom of the cheekbone, easily located by tracing a line along the curve of the cheek and a second down from the eye. This point is often quite tender under pressure, which should be applied upward onto the cheekbone. It can also be helpful for sinus problems and toothache.

NOSEBLEEDS

LI20 (*Yingxiang*) – in the hollow where the nostril meets the cheek. This point needs to be pressed toward the nose with a light touch. **LI20** is also effective for the common cold and nasal congestion.

PC8 (*Laogong*) – in the middle of the palm between the middle and index fingers next to the third metacarpal bone. Press firmly for two to three minutes and repeat on the other hand.

THROAT PROBLEMS

LI14 (*Binao*) – (*see* Toothache, opposite) – helps relieve neck tensions.

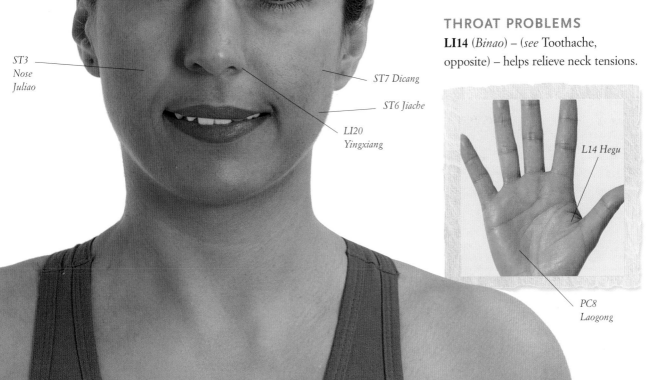

Yintang

ST3 Nose Juliao

ST7 Dicang

ST6 Jiache

LI20 Yingxiang

L14 Hegu

PC8 Laogong

FROZEN SHOULDER

SI10 (*Naoshu*) – on the outer edge of the shoulder blade, just below the joint between the arm and shoulder. This point is often sore to pressure and affects the entire shoulder and neck area.

LOWER BACK PAIN AND SCIATICA

GV6 (*Jizhong*) – just below the eleventh thoracic vertebra. This is best reached with the patient lying face down or bent at the waist, so is difficult for self-administration. Apply gentle pressure with a slight stirring motion. Also effective for sciatica.

Several points on the Urinary Bladder channel can be used in a similar way for lower back pain. They include:

UB23 (*Shenshu*) – level with the space between the second and third lumbar vertebrae

UB57 (*Chengshan*), which is in the hollow in the center of the calf muscle.

UB58 (*Feiyang*) – on the edge of the calf muscle, just below and further out than **UB57**.

UB23 (*Shenshu*) and **UB57** (*Chengshan*) can both be especially effective for the relief of sciatica.

RHEUMATISM

UB15 (*Xinshu*) – level with the fifth thoracic vertebra and one-and-a-half *cun* to the side; press this point firmly with a circular motion for general relief from rheumatic aches and pains in the back.

LI15 (*Jianyu*) – on the hollow or eye on the outside edge of the shoulderbone, felt when the arm is held away from the body. This point can also help pains in the shoulder.

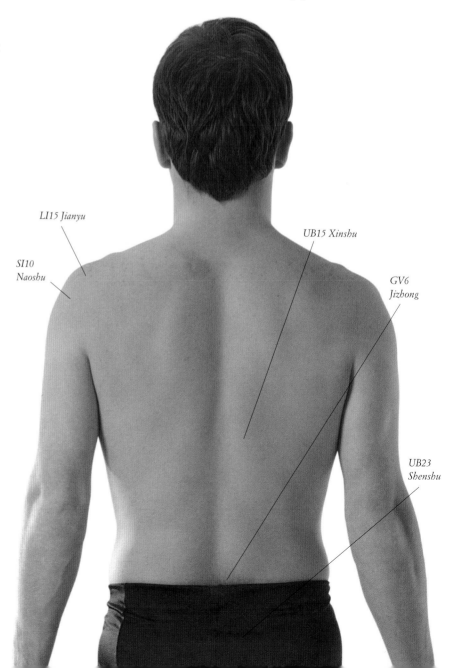

UB57
Chengshan

UB58 Feiyang

LI15 Jianyu

SI10
Naoshu

UB15 Xinshu

GV6
Jizhong

UB23
Shenshu

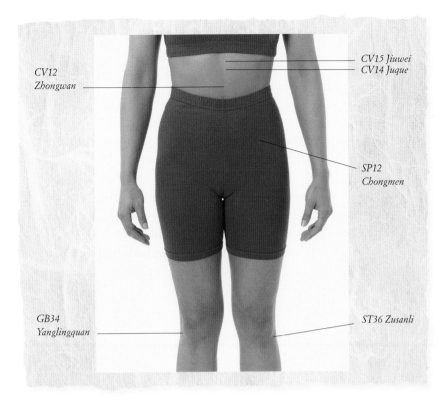

CV15 Jiuwei
CV14 Juque
CV12 Zhongwan
SP12 Chongmen
GB34 Yanglingquan
ST36 Zusanli

CONSTIPATION

GB34 (*Yanglingquan*) – below the top of the fibula (slender leg bone on the outside of the leg), the point can be felt as a slight hollow where the muscles meet just below the knee.

Pressure should be directed toward the inner edge of the fibula. Used to release muscular aches and pains, as well as for various abdominal problems, including constipation and back tension.

SP12 (*Chongmen*) – in the groove between groin and hip bone, about three-and-a-half *cun* to the side of the pubic bone. Apply gentle pressure for two to three minutes.

DIARRHEA

ST25 (*Tianshu*) – two *cun* to the side of the navel (umbilicus). Pressing here can relieve both diarrhea and constipation by normalizing abdominal energy flows.

CV6 (*Qihai*) – one-and-a-half *cun* below the navel on the midline of the abdomen. This point can also be helpful for menstrual problems and for general fatigue – apply pressure with a stirring, circular motion.

FLATULENCE

CV8 (*Shenque*) – center of the navel. Press firmly with a gentle circular motion for two to three minutes.

KD14 (*Siman*) – two *cun* below the navel to one side; the two Kidney meridians on either side of the body are only one *cun* apart here; press fist firmly to cover both points.

INDIGESTION/HEARTBURN

CV15 (*Jiuwei*) – seven *cun* above the navel; press the point on the patient's in-breath using abdominal respiration; release pressure on the out-breath.

CV14 (*Juque*) – six *cun* above the navel; can be used in the same way as **CV15**. Both of these points help in abdominal pain.

UB21 (*Weishu*) – level with the twelfth thoracic vertebra. Press firmly for two to three minutes, with the patient lying on his or her stomach.

NAUSEA

ST36 (*Zusanli*) – (*see* Tired Eyes, page 118). **ST36** should be pressed with a slight stirring motion. This point is also used for abdominal pain.

CV12 (*Zhongwan*) – in the mid-line of the abdomen, four *cun* above the navel. Press firmly with a circular motion.

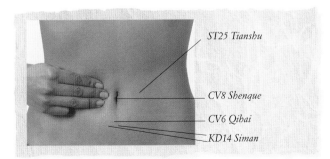

ST25 Tianshu
CV8 Shenque
CV6 Qihai
KD14 Siman

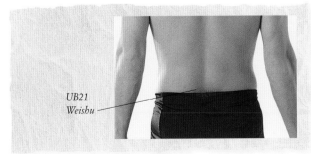

UB21 Weishu

CYSTITIS

LV8 (*Ququan*) – on the inside of the knee, just above the crease produced when the knee is bent. Press gently with a circular motion.

Several points on the Urinary Bladder meridian can also bring relief in cystitis, although these are not quite so accessible for self-administration. Try:

UB18 (*Ganshu*) – one-and-a-half *cun* to the side of the lower border of the ninth thoracic vertebra.

UB27 (*Xiaochangshu*) – in the first depression on the sacrum.

UB28 (*Pangguanshu*) – at the third depression in the sacrum.

UB53 (*Baohuang*) – this is located just outside the top of the sacrum in the dimples of the buttocks, about two *cun* from where the pelvic bone meets the sacrum. This acu point is also helpful for prostate problems, piles, and constipation.

PERIOD PAIN/MENSTRUAL CRAMPS

SP13 (*Fushe*) – almost two *cun* above the middle of the groin inside the lower edge of the pelvic bone. Pressure here can ease any tension in the abdominal area, including menstrual cramps and indigestion.

PREMENSTRUAL SYNDROME

LU8 (*Jingqu*) – in the hollow one *cun* above the wristbone on the thumb side of the arm. The point should be pressed toward the ulna with a light touch.

SP6 (*Sanyinjiao*) – about three *cun* above the ankle bone just behind the edge of the shinbone. Press toward the bone for two to three minutes.

TENSION/STRESS

Easily accessible points like **HT7** (*Shenmen*) are ideal for self-help during fraught periods at work. Lying on a couch while a friend or partner massages the various foot points for you is an ideal way to unwind after a busy day. Among the useful points for stress and tension are:

KD1 (*Yongquan*) – in the depression on the sole, at the ball of the foot. This is a deep point – not surprising, as the flesh here is thickened with walking. Press as hard as possible.

GB18 (*Chengling*) – at the side of the skull – best found by tracing a line diagonally upward from the ear toward the back of the skull, where it intersects with a line passing upward from the neck muscles; the point can be felt as an area of sensitivity.

GB44 (*Foot Qiaoyin*) – on the outside edge of the tip of the fourth toe, nearest to the little toe.

HT7 (*Shenmen*) – on the wrist crease directly below the little finger.

PC8 (*Laogong*) – (*see* Nosebleeds, page 119).

GB34 (*Yanglingquan*) – (*see* Constipation, page 121).

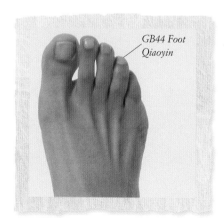

GB44 Foot Qiaoyin

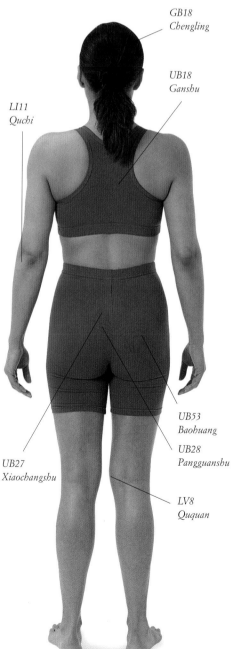

GB18 Chengling

UB18 Ganshu

LI11 Quchi

UB53 Baohuang

UB28 Pangguanshu

UB27 Xiaochangshu

LV8 Ququan

122

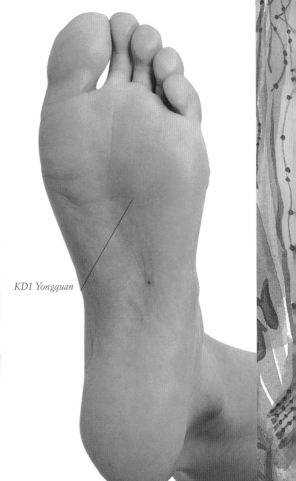

PC6 Neiguan

HT7 Shenmen

LU7 Lieque

PC8 Laogong

FATIGUE

CV4 (*Guanyuan*) – three *cun* below the navel, a warming pressure point for abdominal pain, indigestion, and urinary problems.

PC8 (*Laogong*) – (*see* Nosebleeds, page 119).

CV6 (*Qihai*) – (*see* Diarrhea, page 121).

LI11 (*Quchi*) – in front of the elbow joint, just below the outer crease that is formed when the arm and forearm are bent. This point is also traditionally believed to stimulate the immune system and is used for elbow pain and sprains, fever, and skin problems, as well as depression.

SHOCK

Several points can be used for shock, including:

LU7 (*Lieque*) – about one-and-a-half *cun* above the wrist crease on the thumb side of the inner arm. Gently massage it with a circular motion.

PC6 (*Neiguan*) – on the inner arm, two *cun* above the wrist crease; as well as being helpful for general pain relief, this point is used for dizziness, nausea, and breathing difficulties.

PC9 (*Zhongchong*) – this point can be found on the middle finger at the base of the nail on the side nearest to the forefinger.

GV26 (*Renzhong*) – this is located below the nose, two-thirds of the way above the upper lip.

These four points are all readily accessible, making treatment simpler. Press firmly for two to three minutes.

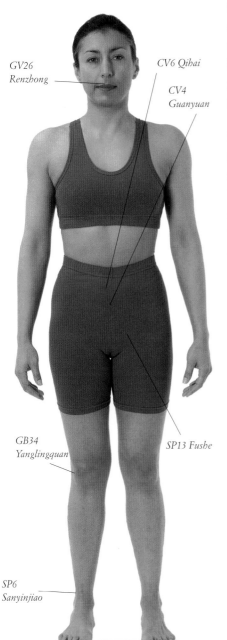

GV26 Renzhong

CV6 Qihai

CV4 Guanyuan

GB34 Yanglingquan

SP13 Fushe

SP6 Sanyinjiao

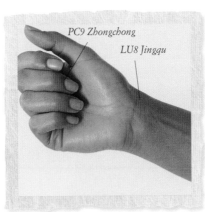

PC9 Zhongchong

LU8 Jingqu

KD1 Yongquan

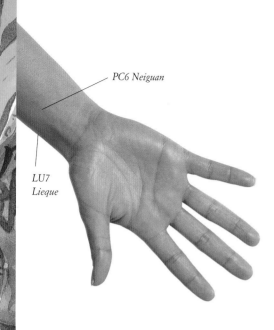

PC6 Neiguan

LU7 Lieque

COMMON COLD

LU7 (*Lieque*) – (*see* Shock, page 123).
GB20 (*Fengchi*)– (*see* Migraine, page 118).

HANGOVER

SP6 (*Sanyinjiao*) – about three *cun* above the ankle bone just behind the edge of the shinbone. Press toward

the bone for two to three minutes. This point can also be helpful for general pain relief and for alleviating premenstrual syndrome.

TRAVEL SICKNESS

Both **PC6** (*Neiguan*) – (*see* Shock, page 123) – and **ST36** (*Zusanli*) – (*see* Tired Eyes, page 118) – are easily accessible when traveling.
Wrist bands designed to put pressure on **PC6** are commercially available in China for travel sickness.
Rather less convenient, although equally effective, is **LV2** (*Xingjian*) – which is located on the web between the first and second toes.
In each case, press the point firmly for two to three minutes with a slight stirring action as you relieve the pressure.

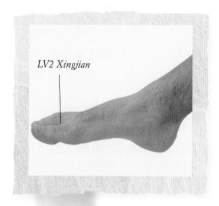

LV2 Xingjian

SPRAINS/SPECIFIC PAINS

NECK

UB10 (*Tianzhu*) – below the base of the skull, a little over one *cun* outward from the center of the neck.
GB20 (*Fengchi*) – (*see* Migraine, page 118) is also helpful.

SHOULDER

GB21 (*Jianjing*) – (*see* Headache, page 118) is also helpful for arthritic problems of the shoulder. Point with a slight circular motion.
LI15 (*Jianyu*) – (*see* Rheumatism, page 120) – this point is also used in China for arthritic shoulder problems as well as strains and sprains.

ELBOW

SJ5 (*Waighuan*) – two *cun* above the crease of the wrist between the arm bones on the back of the wrist.
LI11 (*Quchi*) – (*see* Fatigue, page 123).

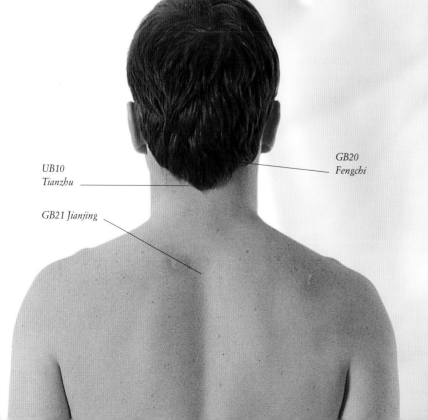

UB10 Tianzhu

GB21 Jianjing

GB20 Fengchi

WRIST

SI4 (*Hand Wangu*) – where the hand joins the arm, in a slight hollow located in the wrist on the ulnar side of the hand.

SI5 (*Yanggu*) – where the hand joins the arm, on the ulnar side edge of the hand, in a depression at the end of the ulna bone.

LI4 (*Hegu*) – (*see* Headache, page 118) can also be helpful for wrist pain.

In each case, press firmly toward the bone.

KNEE

ST35 (*Dubi*) – a point found in the depression below the kneecap when the knee is bent; press firmly toward the kneecap.

Xiyan – one of the extraordinary points found in the depression below the kneecap when the knee is bent – is another useful point to press for knee pains.

UB40 (*Weizhong*) – in the midpoint at the back of the knee between the tendons (*see* back view of figure, page 117). This point is also helpful for pains in the back and thigh – press firmly with a slight circular action.

ANKLE

UB60 (*Kunlun*) – between the ankle and the Achilles tendon on the outside of the ankle, press toward the bone.

ST41 (*Jiexi*) – on the midpoint of the top of the foot between the tendons and in line with the ankle bone.

PAIN

LI4 (*Hegu*) – (*see* Headache, page 118).

PC6 (*Neiguan*) – (*see* Shock, page 123).

SP6 (*Sanyinjiao*) – (*see* Hangover, opposite).

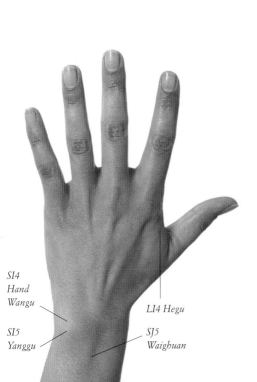

SI4
Hand
Wangu

SI5
Yanggu

LI4 Hegu

SJ5
Waighuan

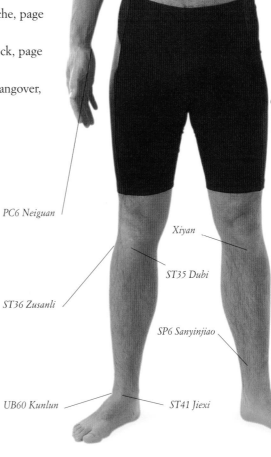

LI11
Quchi

PC6 Neiguan

Xiyan

ST35 Dubi

ST36 Zusanli

SP6 Sanyinjiao

UB60 Kunlun

ST41 Jiexi

THE BREATH OF LIFE

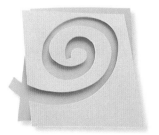

*Q*igong *is one China's oldest forms of therapy, dating back to the days of the Yellow Emperor and the Taoists. Traditionally believed to "eliminate disease and prolong life," it uses exercises that strengthen and focus the* Qi.

LEARNING ENERGY SKILL

Qi is generally translated as "breath" or "vital energy," while *Gong* (or *Gongfu*) can mean the time spent acquiring a skill, the quality of the practice, and the attainment of the art. So *Qigong* may be translated both as "breathing exercise" or "energy skill."

But *Qigong* is more than simply an oriental version of yoga. On one level, it can be a useful form of self-help exercise for improving health and vitality, but it is also an important therapeutic technique. Traditional Chinese hospitals generally have a *Qigong* department where experienced masters teach the technique to patients to help combat chronic diseases like cancer, and they also harness their own *Qi* to use in strengthening massage treatments for the severely ill. *Qigong* healers, for example, can concentrate their energy into their hands which are used to stimulate the paralyzed limbs of stroke patients or brain-damaged babies.

Qigong can also be used as a simple self-help treatment for improving general health and well-being – but it takes practice and dedication or, as the Chinese say, "the most important thing in doing *Qigong* exercise is perseverance."

Qigong exercises are generally divided into three main groups:
• quiescent *Qigong*, which is a type of meditation or "training of the mind"
• dynamic *Qigong*, which focuses on breathing routines or "training the respiration," and
• dynamic–quiescent *Qigong*, which is probably the form most familiar in the West, and includes various postures and movement, or "training of the body."

BELOW **Qi** – the breath of life – is the life force within and all around us.

These different forms can be thought of in terms of yin and yang. Yin can be seen as passive or quiescent (the meditative state); yang can be seen as active or dynamic (the breath). Put them together to make a whole – you have *Qigong*'s dynamic–quiescent postures and movements, where every action is controlled, conscious, and complete.

Timing of *Qigong* exercise is also important and, ideally, needs to match the internal *Qi* clock (*see* pages 28–31). Breathing exercises, for example, should coincide with the

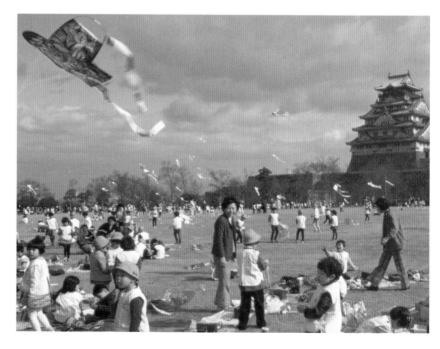

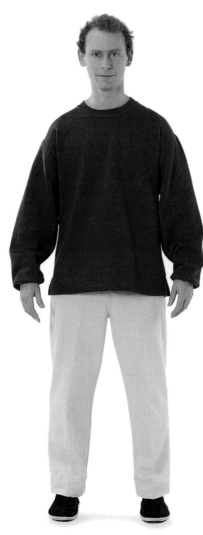

LEFT **Simple
standing in *Qigong*
can involve 18
separate movements.**

time when Lung *Qi* dominates (3 am
to 5 am); this is followed by *Qi* flow
through the associated Large Intestine
(5 am to 7 am). In the spring and
summer, breathing exercises should be
performed at the yin time when
Lung *Qi* dominates, while in the fall
and winter, additional yang is needed
so breathing exercises move to the
yang organ time associated with the
Large Intestine.

QUIESCENT *QIGONG*

Practicing quiescent *Qigong* starts
with a simple standing pose which is
designed to calm the Heart (seat of
the spirit or *Shen* in Chinese theory),
so that you can achieve a peaceful
mind. Simple standing is far from
simple and involves a total of eighteen
separate and conscious movements:

1 The feet should be flat on
the ground, set as wide as your
shoulders, and with the weight
evenly distributed.

2 The knees must be relaxed and
slightly bent so that *Qi* and Blood can
flow freely.

3 The hip joints need to be relaxed.

4 The crotch needs to be slightly
tensed to avoid any leakage of *Qi*
from the "lower door." This is usually
achieved by lifting the kneecaps to
give a lightness to the lower limbs and
then lifting the perineum slightly.

5 The anus is similarly tensed and
lifted in the same way.

6 Tuck in the stomach gently above
the pubic bone to help restrain the
primordial *Qi* and improve *Qi* flow
through the body.

7 The waist must be relaxed to allow
the *Qi* to sink back to the *Dan Tien* –
the area about 5 cm below the navel
and 3 in (7.5 cm) below the surface
that is one of the major areas of the
body where *Qi* is stored. Relaxing the
waist is usually achieved by lifting the
shoulders and then releasing them
downward immediately while
breathing out.

8 The chest must then be pulled in, to
expand the thoracic cavity.

9 Next, the back should be stretched
so that the vertebrae are upright and
the shoulders droop evenly. These
movements calm the Heart and
Lungs, and help the *Ren* and *Du*
channels to communicate.

10 Drooping the shoulder joints also
helps the neck to relax.

11 The elbows are next on the
list – they need to be bent slightly
and then dropped.

12 The elbows then need to be moved
gently away from the body
so that the armpits are open
and hollow.

13 The wrists should be relaxed so
that *Qi* can flow through to the
fingers – this is achieved by gently
hollowing the palm and bending
the fingers.

14 Next, "suspend the head" – best
achieved by imagining it hanging from
a thread so that it is upright and
central to the body.

15 Tuck in the chin.

16 Close the eyes – not tightly but
with eyelids drooping.

17 The lips and teeth need to be
gently closed.

18 Move the tongue so that it is
touching the upper palate. This action
is called "building a bridge" in China,
and forms a link between the *Ren* and
Du channels.

Having achieved this far-from-
simple standing pose, breathe calmly,
clear the mind, and concentrate on the
Dan Tien area. Skilled *Qigong*
exponents will often stand in this way
for several hours focusing on their *Qi*.

> **EXERCISE TIP**
> Try simple standing for five
> minutes to start with.
> Sit down immediately if you
> start to feel faint!

DYNAMIC *QIGONG*

Improving breath control is regarded as an important technique for building *Qi*, since the vital energy is closely associated with the Lungs. By breathing in more and breathing out less, *Qigong* exponents believe they can strengthen inner energies. Unlike passive yoga breathing exercises, *Qigong* breath control is dynamic and involves movement.

The simplest exercise is called "healthy walking" and starts from the standing pose of quiescent *Qigong*. Walk forward with the heel touching the ground and the toes lifted high, while relaxing the head and waist, and swinging the arms gently from side to side so that one hand comes to rest on the *Dan Tien* at the completion of each step.

Look from left and right while walking as if, as the Chinese say, admiring flowers:

> *In flowering shrubs*
> *you walk leisurely*
> *with a smile on your face*
> *and light at heart.*

Breathing should be through the nose – breathing in for two steps and out for one.

CAUTION

If suffering from heart disease or high blood pressure, breathe naturally instead of using *Qigong* breath control

---

DYNAMIC-QUIESCENT *QIGONG*

There are many *Qigong* movement sequences designed to invigorate and strengthen different parts of the body or to combat inherent weaknesses.

Routines can sometimes be less complex than the lengthy *t'ai-chi* cycles and have a clear health focus. The *Baduanjin* or eight silk brocade exercises consist of a series of quite simple movements – only three or four to each stage – which progressively relax the muscles, stretch the limbs and chest, improve the circulation, strengthen the digestive system, nervous system, spine and back, and end with routines to energize the entire body and help concentration.

Other cycles are more lengthy: *Dayan Qigong*, or wild goose *Qigong*, consists of a total of 128 movements that imitate the motion of the wild goose. The first 64 are designed to help postnatal *Qi*, while the second half of the cycle is for prenatal *Qi*. The cycle originated with the Taoists and, like much Taoist therapy, is believed to delay aging and prolong life.

All *Qigong* routines involve an "opening" sequence – activating and moving *Qi* – and then a "closing" cycle to return the invigorated *Qi* to its storage areas. If the exercise is not completed, then the *Qi* can be lost

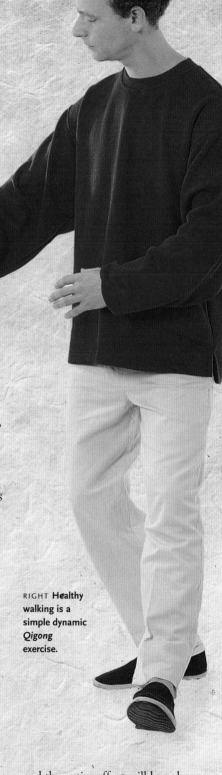

RIGHT **Healthy walking is a simple dynamic *Qigong* exercise.**

and the entire effort will have been wasted. Many books and videotapes are now available giving details of these routines, as well as specialist *Qigong* classes.

DRAWING THE BOW

A typical movement cycle from the eight silk brocade series is "Drawing the Bow." The movements should be performed slowly and deliberately while concentrating on stretching and breathing. This exercise is concentrated on the chest area, helps Blood circulation, and also energizes the arm and shoulder muscles.

1 Start with the simple standing position described earlier.

2 Breathe in, step to the side, and bend the knees as though riding a horse. At the same time, fold your arms across your chest, with your right arm on the outside and your left arm on the inside.

3 With the thumb and forefinger of the left hand extended, and the other three fingers curled together, push out with the left hand while the right hand, tightly clenched, pulls back – as though drawing a bow.

4 Breathe out and return to position 2; breathe in and repeat position 3, but in the opposite direction, extending your right arm.

5 The cycle should be repeated at least ten times, before returning to the standing position once more.

LIFTING ONE ARM

This exercise from the eight silk brocade series is designed to strengthen the digestive system and energize the Liver, Gall Bladder, Spleen, and Stomach.

1 Start from the simple standing position.

2 Breathe in and raise the right arm over the head with the palm up and the fingers pointing to the left, while pressing downward with the left hand, palm down, and the fingers close together, pointing straight ahead.

3 Breathe out and return to the standing position.

4 Repeat position 2, breathing in and raising your left arm and pointing the fingers to the right.

5 Breathe out and return to the standing position.

This exercise should be repeated at least ten times.

ABOVE **Lifting one arm strengthens the digestive system and energizes the abdominal organs.**

RIGHT **Drawing the bow from the** *Baduanjin* **replicates the traditional archer's motion.**

INNER BALANCE FROM *T'AI-CHI*

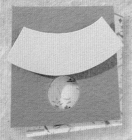

T'ai-chi – *sometimes called* t'ai-chi chu'an – *is one of the many styles of* Qigong *aimed at creating inner harmony. It is often considered to be a Chinese martial art, a type of boxing using both hands and feet to attack the* Qi *of the opponent.*

POSTURE EXERCISES

Like *Qigong, t'ai-chi* is aimed at developing good posture, breath control, and a calm mind – all attributes that are just as essential in meditation as in martial arts. Emphasis in *t'ai-chi* is rather more on posture than on breath control; after all, in any form of hand-to-hand fighting, balance and correct posture will improve defense and attack techniques.

As with other aspects of Chinese medicine, *t'ai-chi* was originally associated with Taoist belief, although it later became more closely linked with the Buddhist Shaolin temples.

Buddhism was brought to China from India during the fifth century by Ta-Mo (Bodhidharma). He used the prevailing form of physical exercise – an early version of *t'ai-chi* – to encourage mental and physical discipline among his followers.

Meditation and a calm mind were essential to them, but the Shaolin monks also gained a reputation for their fighting skills – using *kung fu*. However, they were using fighting, not as an aggressive activity, but as a means of improving physical well-being and therefore spiritual development.

Over the following centuries, Buddhist monks, along with Taoists like Chang San-feng in the 13th century, used *t'ai-chi* as a physical discipline closely associated with spirituality and meditation. Various styles of the exercise evolved, based on these different temple communities.

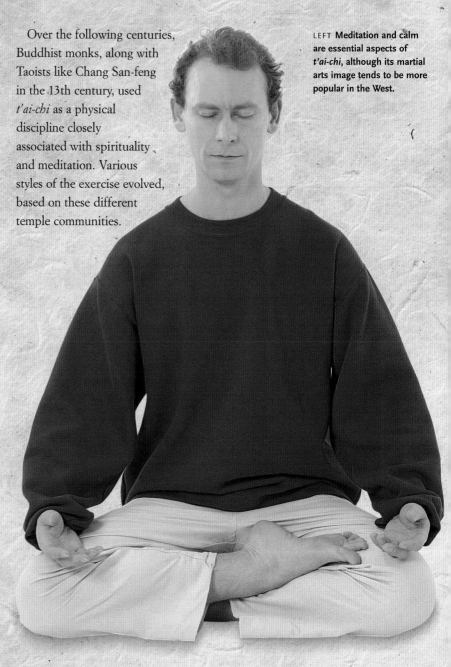

LEFT **Meditation and calm are essential aspects of** *t'ai-chi*, **although its martial arts image tends to be more popular in the West.**

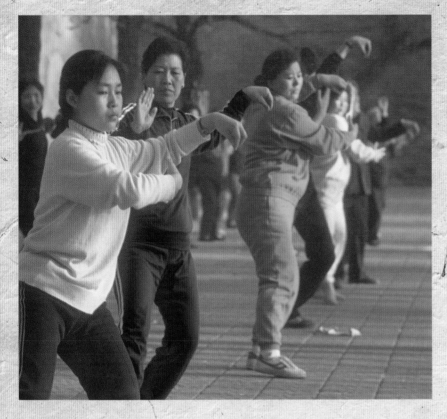

LEFT **Group *t'ai-chi* activity is still a common sight in many parts of China.**

T'AI-CHI GOES UNDERGROUND

In 1644, the Manchurians conquered China and established the Ch'ing dynasty. The new Manchu Emperors knew of the temple traditions of *t'ai-chi* and wanted to learn the skills themselves, so they enlisted Master Yang Lu-chang (1799–1872 CE) to teach them. Master Yang was reluctant to pass on the powerful *Qi*-enhancing skills of *t'ai-chi* to the conquerors, so he reputedly modified the movements to become slow, rather graceful exercise routines, devoid of their inner spirituality.

True *t'ai-chi* he taught only to his sons. This evolved into the Yang family system of *t'ai-chi*, while the elegant exercises practiced by the royal family became a fashionable leisure pursuit for the Chinese aristocracy.

After the revolution of 1900–1910, this leisurely form of *t'ai-chi* spread to the West as *t'ai-chi chu'an* – usually referred to as *t'ai-chi* exercise or Chinese ballet – although *chu'an* or *Quan* actually means fist or boxing. The original temple-style *t'ai-chi* – preserved by generations of the Yang family – has also survived and spread, and is becoming more widely taught in the West as well. Yang-style *t'ai-chi* focuses on *Qi* and developing inner strength, while the *t'ai-chi chu'an* routines are more about balance and stylized fighting techniques.

THE GRAND ULTIMATE

Qi (or *ch'i* in an older system of transliterating Chinese characters) means air, motion, or power. It is usually translated as "vital energy" or "intrinsic energy" with the meaning of "original, eternal, and ultimate energy."

T'ai-chi is considered a harmonious and balanced expression of *Qi*, and is generally translated as "the grand ultimate." Exponents of *t'ai-chi* believe they can transform *Qi* into "internal power" – *Jing* or vital essence – so that, when practicing *t'ai-chi* as a martial art, *Qi* is used to project *Jing* at an opponent. Also important is *Li*, the physical strength or force resulting from body movements. *Li* requires direct physical motion (as in throwing a punch), while *Jing* is an indirect motion – throwing a punch without needing to draw back your fist to gain momentum.

PRACTICING *T'AI-CHI*

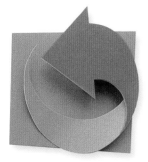

As with Qigong, t'ai-chi *should start with meditation, calming the mind, concentrating on the whole body's natural rhythm and focusing on the* Dan Tien – *an energy center where* Qi *is stored – about 3 in (7.5 cm) below the navel.*

LENGTHY SEQUENCES

As in *Qigong,* numerous styles and sequences of *t'ai-chi* movements are taught, and – also as in *Qigong* – they need to be performed with an alert mind that is focusing on the *Qi.* Sequences can be long, with more than a hundred groups of movements. They are really best taught slowly in a special class with a good teacher. Once you have learned the steps, the whole cycle can be performed quite quickly. While simple *Qigong* motions can quite easily be learned from detailed descriptions in a book, *t'ai-chi* sequences are complicated, and lengthy verbal descriptions inevitably become confusing.

Each motion in the sequences consists of a series of smaller movements that are often very tiny and precise. When learning the sequence, each group of movements is practiced individually several times, and then only gradually integrated into an entire, seamless sequence.

The original Yang sequence, derived from Master Yang Lu-chang, has 108 movements. A shorter form was devised in the 1940s by Cheng Man-ch'ing which has only 37 movements. Other popular styles of *t'ai-chi* taught in the West are known as *Wu, Ch'en, Wudang,* and *Sun.*

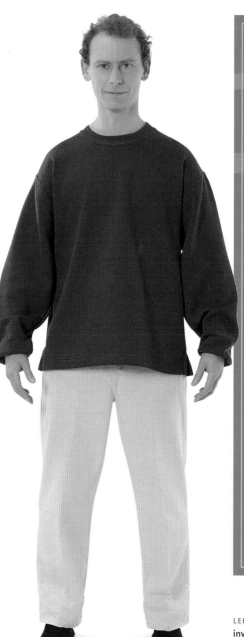

LEFT **Step 1: The beginning form involves simple standing and clearing the mind.**

THE FIVE VIRTUES OF *T'AI-CHI*

1 Your study should be broad and diversified. Do not limit yourself.

2 Examine and question. Ask yourself why *t'ai-chi* works.

3 Be deliberate and careful in your thinking. Use your mind to discover the proper understanding.

4 Clearly examine. Separate concepts distinctly, then decide upon the proper course.

5 Practice sincerely.

Traditional Chinese, translated by Waysun Liao

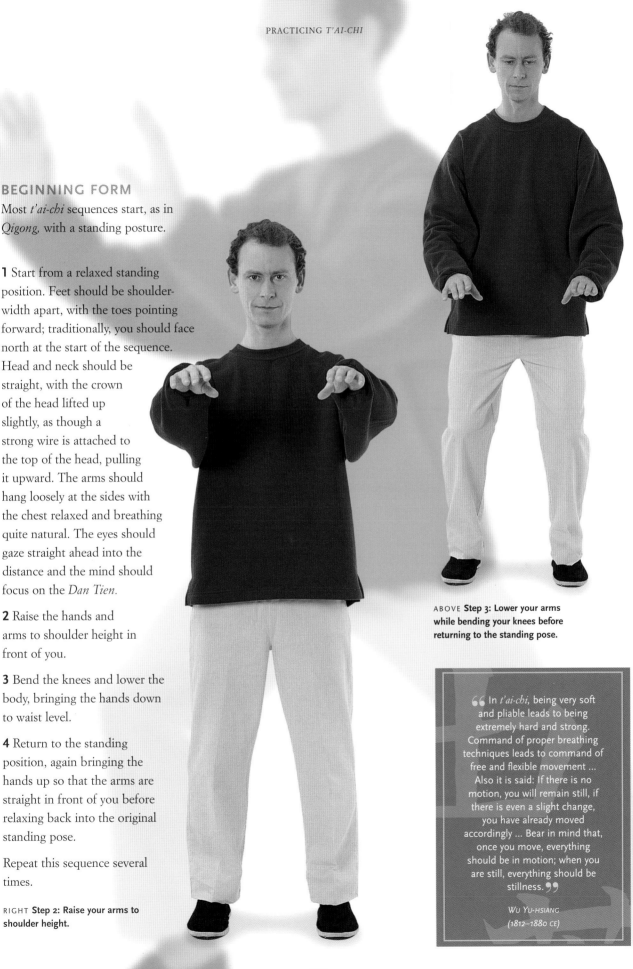

BEGINNING FORM

Most *t'ai-chi* sequences start, as in *Qigong,* with a standing posture.

1 Start from a relaxed standing position. Feet should be shoulder-width apart, with the toes pointing forward; traditionally, you should face north at the start of the sequence. Head and neck should be straight, with the crown of the head lifted up slightly, as though a strong wire is attached to the top of the head, pulling it upward. The arms should hang loosely at the sides with the chest relaxed and breathing quite natural. The eyes should gaze straight ahead into the distance and the mind should focus on the *Dan Tien.*

2 Raise the hands and arms to shoulder height in front of you.

3 Bend the knees and lower the body, bringing the hands down to waist level.

4 Return to the standing position, again bringing the hands up so that the arms are straight in front of you before relaxing back into the original standing pose.

Repeat this sequence several times.

RIGHT **Step 2: Raise your arms to shoulder height.**

ABOVE **Step 3: Lower your arms while bending your knees before returning to the standing pose.**

> In *t'ai-chi*, being very soft and pliable leads to being extremely hard and strong. Command of proper breathing techniques leads to command of free and flexible movement ... Also it is said: If there is no motion, you will remain still, if there is even a slight change, you have already moved accordingly ... Bear in mind that, once you move, everything should be in motion; when you are still, everything should be stillness.
>
> WU YU-HSIANG
> (1812–1880 CE)

T'AI-CHI AND HEALTH

T'ai-chi *encourages flexibility and strength, as well as helping to develop* Qi *and* Jing. *It is also considered to be an excellent method for improving posture.*

It also helps to smooth the flow of *Qi* through the channels and collaterals, clearing any stagnation and blockages. As part of its meditative emphasis, the circular hand movements characteristic of many *t'ai-chi* routines involve imagining the *Qi* as a ball you hold in your hands. At times, it might even be tossed into the air as part of the sequence – but you must be sure, of course, to catch and return your energy by the end of the exercise pattern! With experience, the energy of this *Qi* ball can be felt as a tingling sensation in the hands.

An important part of meditative *t'ai-chi* is to focus the breath on the lower stomach, using the stomach muscles to help the inward and outward flow of air. Chinese practitioners maintain that this sort of movement can help to improve Blood circulation in the abdominal organs (especially the Liver, Kidneys, and Spleen), as well as regulate Heart function. This is due to the movement of the diaphragm; as the stomach pulls air in and pushes it out, it stimulates the nerves in the lower spine.

ABOVE **Many t'ai-chi exercises involve visualizing the Qi as a ball of energy.**

BREATH CONTROL
Although *t'ai-chi* is regarded by many as a martial art, it really belongs, because of its links with *Qigong*, with health therapies. As a martial art, it was intended to develop balance and strength, and the emphasis is on posture and upright positions – with that string always pulling on the crown of the head.

GRASP THE BIRD'S TAIL
The names of movements are often graphic descriptions of the actions involved. This sequence is known as "grasp the bird's tail" or "grasp the sparrow's tail." Start in the original standing pose (*see* page 127). Stretch your right arm out, palm facing up, and move it upward. Put all your weight on your right foot, moving your left foot beside your right foot. Bring your left palm down and bend your right elbow until your palms are facing each other.

1 Take a step with your left foot, putting your heel to the floor first. At the same time, start to stretch out your left forearm and bring down your right hand. Move your weight forward as you finish these arm movements.

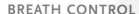

1

134

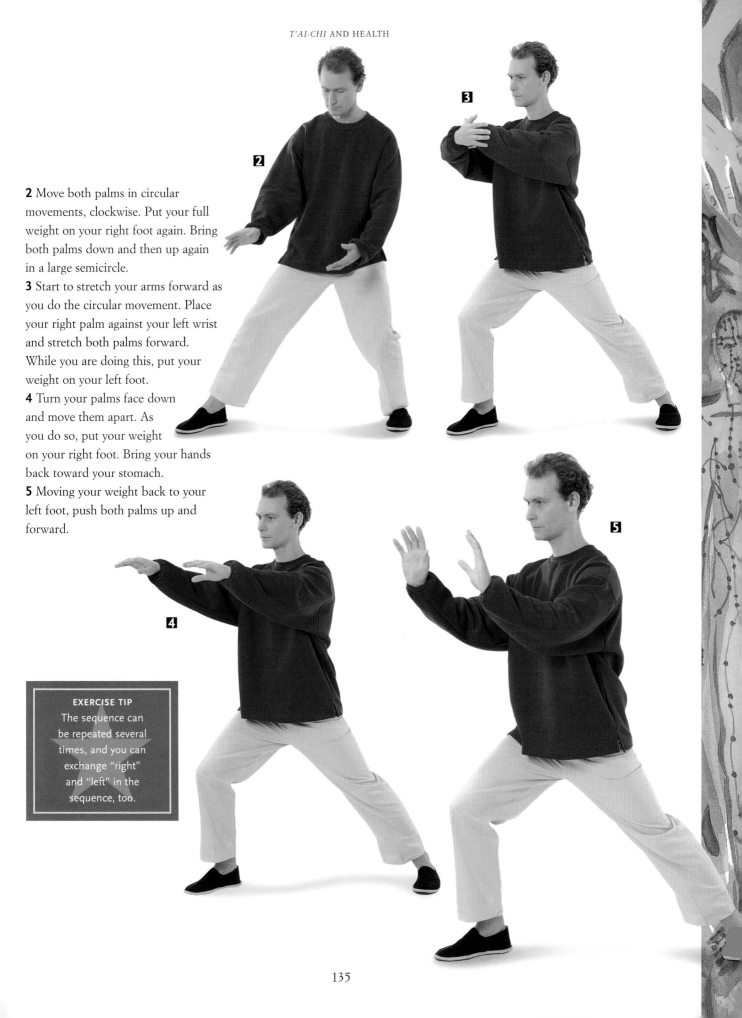

2 Move both palms in circular movements, clockwise. Put your full weight on your right foot again. Bring both palms down and then up again in a large semicircle.

3 Start to stretch your arms forward as you do the circular movement. Place your right palm against your left wrist and stretch both palms forward. While you are doing this, put your weight on your left foot.

4 Turn your palms face down and move them apart. As you do so, put your weight on your right foot. Bring your hands back toward your stomach.

5 Moving your weight back to your left foot, push both palms up and forward.

EXERCISE TIP
The sequence can be repeated several times, and you can exchange "right" and "left" in the sequence, too.

GLOSSARY

ACUPRESSURE Chinese healing therapy designed to rebalance or unblock the flow of energy within the body. Pressure is used at certain points on the body, which correspond to points on the meridians

ACU POINTS Specific points on the body where the energy flow through the body meridians can be adjusted

ARTHRITIS Painful inflammation of joint tissues

ASTHMA Spasm of the bronchi in the lungs, narrowing the airways

AURICULAR Pertaining to the ear

BRONCHITIS Inflammation of the bronchi, the tubes that take air to the lungs

CHANNELS Invisible pathways in which *Qi* travels; also called **meridians**. They appear in and on the body

CHONG MAI The penetrating vessel; one of the eight extraordinary meridians

CONTRAINDICATION Any factor in a patient's condition that indicates that a treatment would be inappropriate and is therefore not recommended

CUPPING A treatment technique involving drawing the *Qi* and blood to the surface of the skin using a vacuum created inside a glass or bamboo cup

DAI MAI The girdle vessel; one of the eight extraordinary meridians

DAMP In Chinese medicine, Damp is considered to be a yin pathogenic influence, leading to sluggishness, tired and heavy limbs and general lethargy

DAN TIEN Energy centers in the body. In Chinese medicine there are considered to be three; an upper (between the eyebrows); a middle (in the center of the trunk); and a lower (in the lower abdomen). *Qi* is considered as being stored there

DECOCTION A herbal preparation, where the plant material is boiled in water and reduced to make a concentration extract

DEFICIENT CONDITION One where there is a lack of basic constituents (i.e. *Qi*, Blood, or Body Fluids) or where there is inadequate function of any *Zang Fu* organ

DU MAI The governing vessel; one of the eight extraordinary meridians

EDEMA A painless swelling caused by fluid retention

EIGHT PRINCIPLE PATTERNS The system of organizing diagnostic information in Chinese medicine according to the principles of yin, yang; Interior, Exterior; Hot, Cold; Excess, Deficiency

EXCESS CONDITION One where there is a surplus or congestion of basic constituents (i.e. *Qi*, Blood or Body Fluids) or where there is inadequate function of any *Zang Fu* organ

EXTERNAL In Chinese medicine, any factors influencing the body from outside

FIVE ELEMENTS The system in Chinese medicine based on observations of the natural world. The system is built around the elements of water, wood, fire, metal, and earth

FU The hollow yang organs of the body

HOLISTIC Aiming to treat the individual as an entity, incorporating body, mind, and spirit

HYPERTENSION Raised blood pressure

INTERNAL In Chinese medicine, it refers to aspects of disharmonies that arise within the body

JIN-YE Body Fluids; Jin refers to the lighter fluids, Ye to the denser fluids

JING The vital essence that is the source of life and invidual development

MARROW The substance that makes up the brain and spinal column in Chinese medicine

MATERIA MEDICA Substances used in medicine; the science of their properties and use

MERIDIANS The channels through which vital energy flows in the body. In Chinese acupuncture, there are 59 meridians in all (12 main ones)

MOXA Dried mugwort, which is burned on the end of needles, or rolled into a stick and then heated in moxabustion treatment. It is said to warm the *Qi* in the body, in order to increase its flow

MOXABUSTION The treatment approach involving the burning of the herb, **moxa**

MUCUS Slimy fluid secreted by various membranes in the body

PHLEGM In Chinese medicine, Disharmony of the Body Fluids produces either external (visible) Phlegm, or internal (invisible) Phlegm

QI The Chinese term for the life force or vital energy of the universe, which is fundamental to all aspects of life. It permeates the whole body and is concentrated in the channels

QIGONG A series of moving and static exercises associated with the breath

REN MAI The conception vessel; one of the eight extraordinary meridians

SAN JIAO Triple burner or triple heater – a manifestation of the process of digestion sometimes included with the Zang organs

SHEN Spirit, a fundamental substance and expression of the life force; one of the "three treasures" of Chinese medicine, seen in the brightness of the eyes

T'AI-CHI A form of exercise and meditational practice commonly associated in the West with martial arts

TANG Soup: a traditional decoction and method of taking herbs

TAO/TAOISM Chinese philosophical and spiritual system. *Tao* literally means "the way"

THREE TREASURES The collective term used to describe *Qi, Jing,* and *Shen*

TINCTURE A herbal remedy prepared in an alcohol base

TONIFICATION A process in Chinese medicine that involves strengthening the Blood and *Qi*

WEI QI Defensive *Qi,* which protects the body from invasion by external pathogenic factors. It flows just beneath the skin

XUE The Chinese term for Blood

YANG One aspect of the complementary opposites in Chinese philosophy. Reflects the more active, moving, warmer aspects; *see also* yin

YIN One aspect of the complementary opposites in Chinese philosophy. Reflects the more passive, reflective, cooler aspects; *see also* yang

ZANG The solid yin organs of the body

ZANG FU The term used in traditional Chinese medicine for the complete yin and yang organs of the body (different from those of Western anatomy)

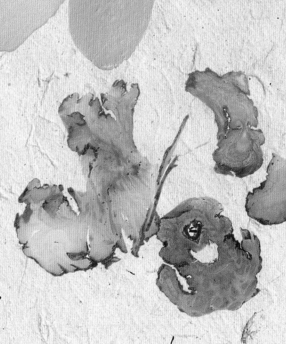

USEFUL ADDRESSES

AUSTRALIA

*Australian Natural
Therapists Association*
PO Box 308
Melrose Park 5039
South Australia
Tel +61 8 297 9533
Fax +61 8 297 0003

*Australian Traditional
Medicine Society Limited*
(Mailing)
ATMS
PO Box 1027
Meadowbank
NSW 2114
Tel +61 2 809 6800

(Office)
ATMS
12/27 Bank Street
Meadowbank
NSW 2114

Qigong Association of Australia
458 White Horse Road
Surrey Hills
Victoria 3127
Tel +61 3 9836 6961
Fax +61 3 830 5608

UNITED KINGDOM

British Acupuncture Association
34 Alderney Street
London
SW1V 4EU

British Acupuncture Council
Park House
206–208 Latimer Road
London W10 6RE
Tel +44 181 964 0222
Fax +44 181 964 0333

*British Complementary
Medicine Association*
39 Prestbury Road
Cheltenham
Gloucestershire GL52 2PT
Tel +44 1242 226770
Fax +44 1242 226778

*British Council for
Chinese Martial Arts*
28 Linden Farm Drive
Countesthorpe
Leicester LE8 5SX
Tel/Fax +44 116 2774260

East West Herbs Ltd
Langston Priory Mews
Kingham
Oxon OX7 6UW

*National Institute of Medical
Herbalists*
56 Longbrook Street
Exeter
Devon EX4 6AH

Register of Chinese Herbal Medicine
PO Box 4000
Wembley
Middlesex HA9 9NZ
Tel +44 181 904 1357

Tai Chi Union for Great Britain
102 Felsham Road
London SW15 1DQ

UNITED STATES

*American Association of
Oriental Medicne (AAOM)*
433 Front Street
Catasauqua
PA 18032
Tel +1 610 2661433
Fax +1 610 2642768

*The Chi Kung School at
The Body-Energy Center*
James MacRitchie
and Damaris Jarboux
PO Box 19708
Boulder
CO 80308
Tel +1 303 4422250
Fax +1 303 4423141

*The International Chi Kung/
Qi Gong Directory*
PO Box 19708
Boulder
CO 80308
Tel +1 303 4423131
Fax +1 303 4423141

*National Accreditation Commission for
Schools and Colleges of Acupuncture
and Oriental Medicine (NACSCAOM)*
1010 Wayne Avenue
Suite 1270
Silver Springs
MD 20910
Tel +1 301 6089680
Fax +1 301 6089576

*National Acupuncture and Oriental
Medicine Alliance (National Alliance)*
14637 Starr Road, SE
Olalla
WA 98359
Tel +1 206 8516896
Fax +1 206 8516883

*National Commission for the
Certification of Acupuncturists (NCCA)*
PO Box 97075
Washington DC 20090-7075
Tel +1 202 2321404
Fax +1 202 4626157

Qigong Academy
8103 Marlborough Avenue
Cleveland
OH 44129
Tel/Fax +1 408 4760665

FURTHER READING

BEINFIELD, H., and KORNGOLD, E. (1991) *Between Heaven and Earth,* Ballantine Books, New York.

BENSKY. D., and GAMBLE, A. (1986) *Chinese Herbal Medicine,* Eastland Press, Seattle

BLOFIELD, J. (1978) *Taoism: The Road to Immortality,* Shambhala, Boston.

BONE, K. (1996) *Clinical Applications of Ayurvedic and Chinese Herbs,* Phytotherapy Press, Queensland.

COOPER, J. C. (1981) *Yin and Yang,* Aquarian Press, Northampton.

CHIN, W. Y., and KENG, H, (1990) *An Illustrated Dictionary of Chinese Medicinal Herbs,* CRCS Publications, Sebastapol. Ca.

DONG, T. P. (1993) *Still as a Mountain, Powerful as Thunder,* Shambhala, Boston.

FLAWS, B., and WOLFE, H. (1983) *Prince Wen Hui's Cook: Chinese Dietary Therapy,* Paradigm Publications, Brookline, Ma

FOSTER, S., and YUE, C. (1992) *Herbal Emissaries,* Healing Arts Press, Rochester, VT.

FULDER, S. (1982) *The Tao of Medicine,* Destiny Books, New York.

HIEP, N. D. (1987) *The Dictionary of Acupuncture and Moxabustion,* Thorsons, Northampton.

HOBBS, C. (1995) *Medicinal Mushrooms,* Botanica Press, Santa Cruz.

HOIZEY, D. and M.-J. (tr, Bailey P.) (1993) *A History of Chinese Medicine,* Edinburgh University Press.

HSIUNG, D.-T. (1999) *The Chinese Kitchen,* Kyle Cathie, London

HUI, J. L., and XIANG, J. Z. (1986) *Pointing Therapy,* Shandong Science and Technology Press.

HUYNH, H. K. (tr.) (ed. G. M. Siefert) (1981). *Li Shi Zhen's Classic Pulse Diagnosis,* Paradigm Publications, Brookline, Ma.

HYATT, R. (1978) *Chinese Herbal Medicine,* Thorsons, New York.

KAPTCHUK, T. (1983) *Chinese Medicine: The Web that has No Weaver,* Rider, London

LEUNG, A. Y. (1985) *Chinese Herbal Remedies,* Wildwood House, London.

LEWITH, G. T. (1082) *Acupuncture,* Thorsons, Northampton.

LIU, Y. (1988) *The Essential Book of Traditional Chinese Medicine,* Colombia University Press, New York.

LU, H. C. (1986) *Chinese System of Food Cures,* Sterling Publishing, New York

MACIOCIA, G. (1987) *Tongue Diagnosis in Chinese Medicine,* Eastland Press, Seattle.

MILLS, S. Y. (1991) *Out of the Earth,* Viking, London.

ODY, P. (1993) *The Herb Society's Complete Medicinal Herbal,* Dorling Kindersley, London.

SANDIFER, J. (1997) *Acupressure,* Element, Shaftesbury.

TAKAHASHI, M., and BROWN, S. (1986) *Qigong for Health,* Japan Publications, New York.

TANG, S., and CRAZE, R. (1995) *Chinese Herbal Medicine,* Piatkus, London.

TEEGUARDEN, R. (1985) *Chinese Tonic Herbs,* Japan Publications, New York.

VEITH, I. (ed.) (1966) *The Yellow Emperor's Classic of Internal Medicine,* University of California Press.

WILLARD, T. (1990) *Reishi Mushroom,* Sylvan Press, Washington.

YANG, J.-M. (1988) *The Eight Pieces of Brocade,* Yang's Martial Arts Association, Massachusetts.

YANG, S.-Z. (tr.) (1998) *The Divine Farmer's Materia Medica,* Blue Poppy Press, Boulder, Co.

YEN, K.-Y. (1992) *The Illustrated Chinese Materia Medica,* SMC Publishing, Taipei.

YEUNG, H.-C. (1985) *Handbook of Chinese Herbs and Formulas,* Institute of Chinese Medicine, Los Angeles.

ZHEN, C.X. (1985) *The Massotherapy of Traditional Chinese Medicine,* Hai Feng Publishing, Hong Kong.

ZHONG, M. (tr. Zhang, K.) (1986) *The Chinese Plum-Blossom Needle Therapy,* The People's Medicinal Publishing House, Beijing

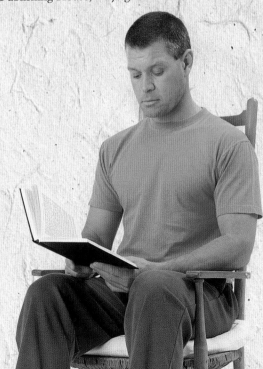

INDEX

Acknowledgements

The publishers wish to thank the following for the use of pictures:

Art Directors & Trip: Ask, p.99; J. Highet, p.86; A. Tovy, p.33t; P. Treanor, p.53tl; M. Watson, p.87

Corbis: Horace Bristol, p.93l; Jack Fields, p.126; Wolfgang Kaehler, p.131; Earl Kowall, p.94b; Phil Schermeister, p.54tr

The Image Bank: Chuck Kuhn, p.12tl; D. Redfearn, p.12t; Michael Salas, pp.5 and 12bl; Thomas Schmitt, p.12tr

Harry Smith Collection: pp.74tc and 83tl

Tony Stone Images: Chave/Jennings, pp.1 and 57; Andy Cox, pp.24–25b; Margaret Gowan, pp.110–111b; Pat Hermansen, p.33b; Zigy Kaluzny, p.89; Yann Layma, p.37; Laurence Monneret, pp.25tr and 31tr; Les Wies, pp.54–55

Superstock: Paul Kuroda, p.35b

Key: b = bottom; c = center; l = left; r = right; t = top

Special thanks go to **East West Herbs**, Kingham, Oxfordshire, UK, for help with properties